THE SERVICE LINE SOLUTION

Consumer-Focused Strategies for the Accountable Care Era

E. Preston Gee

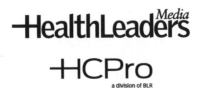

a division of BLR

E. Preston Gee, Author
Claudette Moore, Acquisitions Editor
Erin Callahan, Senior Director, Product
Doug Ponte, Cover Designer
Michael McCalip, Graphic Designer/Layout
Matt Sharpe, Production Supervisor

Advice given is general. Readers should consult professional counsel for specific legal, ethical, or clinical questions.

Arrangements can be made for quantity discounts. For more information, contact:

HCPro
75 Sylvan Street, Suite A-101
Danvers, MA 01923
Telephone: 800/650-6787 or 781/639-1872
Fax: 800/639-8511
Email: *customerservice@hcpro.com*

Visit HCPro online at:
www.hcpro.com and *www.hcmarketplace.com*

Contents

About
the Author

E. Preston Gee

E. Preston Gee is the Vice President of Strategic Marketing for CHRISTUS Health in Dallas, Texas. He is a recognized thought leader in the healthcare industry, particularly in the areas of consumer-driven healthcare, service line strategy, and most recently on the topic of health insurance exchanges/marketplaces. His professional experience includes senior executive positions with some of the largest nonprofit and for-profit health systems in the nation.

Over the course of his career, Gee has published numerous articles on planning and strategy for virtually every major publication in the healthcare industry. He is a frequent speaker on consumer-based trends and market-facing strategy. *The Service Line Solution* is Gee's tenth professional book. Gee began his career in the packaged-goods industry with The Quaker Oats Company/Fisher-Price Toys Division. He holds B.S and MBA degrees from Brigham Young University in Provo, Utah, and is a past recipient of the *Modern Healthcare* "Up and Comer's Award."

Foreword

Why Service Lines Are the Solution

The healthcare industry is undergoing what may be the most significant change in more than 40 years. Much of the upheaval is due to the sweeping impact of healthcare reform (especially the implementation of insurance exchanges), but the change is most certainly a result of market momentum as well.

The convergence of government legislation and market dynamics have driven virtually everyone in the industry to rethink and revisit their central business strategy. However, far too few executives recognize that optimizing service line (SL) architecture and strategy is one of the most viable and effective responses to the demands of the Affordable Care Act and the focus on population health.

While some may scoff at the notion that SL strategy is the key to addressing such sweeping changes, even the most ardent skeptics can't ignore market conditions that align with the SL construct. Among these are:

- Increased *financial engagement* on the part of the patient/consumer, in the form of increased copays, deductibles, and percentage of the overall insurance premium.

- Mounting influence of the Internet and the resulting *empowerment of the patient/consumer,* who has unlimited access to disease-specific information and therefore relies less on medical professionals for education.

- Heightened *emphasis on value* of provided services, resulting from greater transparency regarding the costs and correlating quality of those services.

- Rising pressure on traditional providers related to *pricing and convenient access* from consumer-savvy enterprises like big-box stores (e.g., Wal-Mart) and retail pharmacies (e.g., CVS and Walgreens).

Keep in mind that the forces listed above began building prior to the advent of health insurance exchanges, a development that most industry pundits agree will have an accelerating impact on the "consumerization" of healthcare. All of this argues for a renewed emphasis on SL strategy as the solution to meet the current and expected changes in the health sector.

In essence, we are facing a time that industry strategy and marketing experts have long anticipated: when healthcare will begin to look like most other industries in this nation, driven by market forces and consumer interests.

For that reason and others that will be explored in this book, the SL approach is the optimal architecture for effectively meeting the emerging demands of the healthcare/medical marketplace.

Strategists, Marketing Mavens, and Why They Matter

So you might be asking, if an SL strategy overhaul is the best tool for addressing the dramatic changes facing our industry, why don't we hear more about it, and why aren't more organizations moving in that direction?

Allow me a moment of brutal candor: Many healthcare executives in hospital and health system settings do not fully understand the principles of marketing. This rather bold assessment isn't meant to cast aspersions on senior healthcare executives, many of whom have obviously done quite well in the industry, thank you very much. No, the fact is that healthcare from the provider vantage has not required or even lent itself to an understanding of fundamental marketing practices.

The meaning of "market-driven"

No matter what the pundits say, healthcare in this nation has never really been market-driven. How could it be when the vast majority of its consumers (patients) see (and pay) only a small fraction of the total costs of the services rendered? For the private sector (commercial health insurance) as well as the government-financed area (Medicare and Medicaid), total costs are camouflaged in complex billing practices and consequently are not a driving factor for consumers. Therefore, anyone who maintains that we should keep the industry "market driven" is either pushing an agenda or not familiar with market-driven industries.

When I moved from the packaged-goods industry to healthcare nearly three decades ago, I was struck by how little this sector applied general marketing practices to its underlying strategies. At first, I was perplexed, then frustrated, and finally irritated. Then I had the epiphany: *Of course* executives in this field don't apply the concepts we learned in business school as related to the marketing function. This industry is an anomaly—and not only from a *financial accountability* standpoint. Healthcare is also the exception with regard to *access* and applicable industry knowledge. What other industry offers its services—by legal mandate—to those who can't pay for them?

In addition, what other industry has fundamentally "protected" the basic understanding of its services with such rigor and effectiveness over the decades? Let's face it: The recent movement toward transparency in healthcare, although valuable and welcome, is relatively new—and due in large part to the Internet.

Decades ago, in his seminal book, *The Socialization of American Medicine*, Paul Starr observed that "Not only did physicians become a powerful, prestigious, and wealthy profession, but they succeeded in shaping the basic organization and financial structure of American medicine…" In short, the medical profession's well-protected complexity and seeming cognitive impenetrability produced a dependent public that relied unquestioningly on the expertise of licensed professionals, specifically on the physicians who treated them. That is not exactly the kind of dynamic that's conducive to market forces, at least not when compared to virtually every other industry in America, where the consumer has extensive access not only to the nature of goods or services provided but to the design, delivery, and financing process as well.

Given the financial disconnect between patient and the true *cost* of care, and the absence of information providing a *value* measurement (i.e., quality of care provided relative to the cost of the services rendered), no wonder healthcare marketing was discounted or in some cases ignored altogether. Today, the barriers to informed decisions are breaking down, and meaningful change is upon us. The link between accountability and payment is more accessible than ever. Increasingly engaged and knowledgeable consumers/patients finally have the tools to assess "value" and to make healthcare financing decisions accordingly.

Advice from Someone Who's Been There

One might ask, why another book on service lines, and particularly, why another one from Preston Gee? Good questions, to which the answers are: expertise and timing. As noted above, I migrated from the packaged-goods industry to the health sector nearly three decades ago, just as marketing and strategic planning were starting to emerge in the hospital and health system world. I made an industry-changing move from Quaker Oats/Fisher-Price Toys to Sacred Heart

Hospital in Eugene, Oregon, part of the Sisters of St. Joseph of Peace system, now Peace Health. The fellow who hired me, Jim Folger, had worked for the Heinz Corporation. We were both new to healthcare but familiar with product-line management, thanks to our previous employers. Therein lies the expertise part of the equation.

Jim and I decided to apply some of our background—*and expertise*—in packaged/consumer goods to the managerial structure of marketing and strategy. Eventually, we decided to commit that perspective to paper for a broader audience. We co-authored *Product Management for Hospitals: Organizing for Profitability,* the first book on product-line management for healthcare, which became known as service line management in the early to mid-nineties. At the time, we thought the principles and practices that had worked so well for a vast array of consumer-facing industries would apply to healthcare as well. To a certain extent, they did.

At that time, the conditions for a product/SL structure were not as favorable in the healthcare industry as they had been in more market-driven industries. However, that is about to change—and is already changing—with the advent of insurance exchanges and the sweeping momentum of the market toward a more consumer-based landscape. And that's where the timing part comes in.

To paraphrase Ralph Waldo Emerson, who famously observed, "This time, like all times, is the best of times," this time is definitely the best of times for a managerial framework that aligns progressive organizations closely with their most important stakeholder: the consumer. I use the term "consumer" here deliberately, and not consumer/patient (as will be referenced several times throughout the book), to emphasize the shift we are seeing and will continue to see toward a consumer-driven environment.

This dramatic shift will be even more pronounced under accountable care and population health. By necessity, we must shift our focus from the patient who is treated episodically to the consumer who is educated and empowered holistically, hopefully receiving care in the most appropriate and efficient setting ... or not receiving care at all. But much more on that later.

For now, the important thing to keep in mind is that your retooled SL strategy will be a requirement of the post-ACA environment; the market will demand it, and consumers will embrace it. And who better to guide you and your organization through these uncharted waters than a former consumer-goods guy, who has been advocating for and writing about SL structure and strategy for nearly three decades?

As they say, timing—*and experience*—are everything.

Preston Gee

Introduction

The Service Line Solution is intended to provide a comprehensive guide to the key elements of service line management (SLM) in a rapidly changing healthcare industry. The strategies in this book are sharply trained on the convergence of two key market factors: a move toward a more consumer-focused orientation, and the emergence of population health management as the means to effectively manage defined populations. In this book, you'll find the key steps necessary to develop an effective SL architecture for hospitals and health systems, presented in sequence and designed with the idea that the new environment we face will require not only a modified structure but also a dramatically different approach to this consumer-empowered world.

In that regard, the first four chapters of the book provide background on the SL structure and the rationale for this approach, which has been so effectively utilized in virtually all other industries in America, is more applicable and germane to healthcare than ever before. This part of the book also addresses significant changes that have occurred in SLM since the precursor to this book, *Service Line Execution 2.0,* was written seven years ago.

These early chapters speak definitively to the migration to a consumer-driven landscape and why that seismic shift requires a different mind-set on the part of hospital and health system leaders. This shift is significant, since healthcare in the United States has not experienced the kind of market-oriented dynamics that most other sectors of the national economy have witnessed. However, few leading organizations in the field are effectively transitioning to a model that is more retail than wholesale oriented.

Chapter 3 specifically provides background and thematic rationale for why the industry is in its most serious state of flux in several decades; namely the advent and actualization of insurance exchanges. As this chapter points out, irrespective of the political implications of exchanges, the undeniable reality is that this emerging market force–either in the public or private sector–engages the patient/consumer to a much greater degree and empowers them in a way that has not existed in healthcare since its inception. The purpose of this chapter is to provide context and the conceptual framework for addressing these shifting dynamics. Chapter 4 looks at the impact of population health on the SL application and specifically speaks to why an SL structure is invaluable for implementing an effective population health model.

Chapters 5 through 11 outline the basic framework of an SL structure and the steps to either developing or enhancing SL architecture. Included in this group of chapters are elements such as the need for data-based definitions, the value of using quantifiable metrics as the basis for assessing performance, the imperative to narrow the number of SLs down to a manageable core (no more than four at the outset), and the role of the SL manager in effectively marshaling the resources and focus of the organization to achieve competitive differentiation. Chapter 11 focuses on the inherent value of disciplined business planning and includes a discussion regarding the value of market research in gauging consumer perception and competitive advantage.

The final two chapters, Chapter 12 and Chapter 13, delve into execution and explore the need to manage SLs much like strategic business units, with extensive analytics and a competitive thrust. This section also addresses second-stage implementation of an SL structure, by adding additional SLs to the mix once the organization has effectively implemented the original two to four core SLs.

1

The
Service Line
Moment

Retooling Our Service Line Strategies for New Realities

As we move from patient-centered healthcare to the consumer-based model
triggered by health insurance exchanges, the locus of control is shifting to
individual consumers, away from professional practitioners and the institutions
that support them. And that is nothing short of a seismic shift.

Yet few healthcare organizations have taken critical steps to retool their service
line management (SLM) models for the post-Affordable Care Act (ACA) world.
Only the most progressive have rethought the SLM construct to address the
convergence of two sweeping movements in our industry: population health
management and rising consumer engagement.

While many industry advisors have recognized the individual impact that each
movement will have on the healthcare landscape, only a small percentage have

grasped the significance of the junction of these powerful market dynamics. The two major movements, in fact, are rarely discussed in the same conversation.

Although the "imminent rise of the consumer" has been predicted for a couple of decades, what makes this time different is the impact of exchanges (or marketplaces, as they are sometimes called) coupled with the individual consumer's economic responsibility. In addition, the goal under an accountable care model will often be to keep the consumer/patient out of the hospital and directed to more appropriate and less-expensive care venues.

These critical factors will finally engage the gears of the market in a way we've only dreamed of in the past.

Old thinking—the passive patient

The reasons that so many fail to see the strategic linkage between population health and consumer empowerment are many, but, fundamentally, it comes down to old thinking. The traditional mind-set in healthcare—that the patient is basically a "receiver" of services provided—is deeply entrenched and is still a predominant perception.

The consumer as a passive recipient of services is unheard of in virtually every other industry in America. Usually, consumers are acknowledged to be the driving factor in the development and design of those services. The role of the healthcare consumer is changing, and that shift will play a pivotal role in altering our industry.

The move to population health alone won't reshape the image of patients as simple service receivers, however. Population health (which is somewhat of a misnomer, but more on that later) is primarily being interpreted from the traditional view of healthcare design and delivery; many experts have not yet put the proactive consumer at the center of their strategies for addressing population health and delivery of accountable care.

That is an unfortunate and arguably provincial view.

New reality—the active consumer

Healthcare in America is changing more rapidly than it ever has in the history of the industry. Costs continue to rise at a rapid clip, but more important than the overall cost index figures is the cost impact on the individual. People at all stages of life and in all sectors of the work force are paying more for their share of the healthcare pie through increased deductibles, copayments and monthly premiums—that is if they're fortunate to have an employer that offers health insurance.

Those without health insurance know first-hand the sharp sting of medical bills, an often-untenable financial burden at the core of more than half of the personal bankruptcies in the country. The clamor for a solution to this nationwide dilemma was a primary factor in the successful passage of the Affordable Care Act (ACA), colloquially termed "Obamacare." The cornerstone of the ACA was actualized in 2014 with the implementation of health insurance exchanges, following an infamously rugged enrollment ramp-up due to technical glitches.

Regardless of one's political views, however, the reality is that the ACA shifts control away from the traditional power brokers and influential stakeholders. It shifts power to a newly engaged consumer, who is more economically responsible and therefore a more conscientious purchaser of the services offered.

The Service Line Advantage

The underlying promise of this book is simple: By executing on a consumer-optimized SL strategy, you will successfully meet the complex demands of an accountable care environment **and** streamline your approach for a world in which the engaged consumer is—as the adage goes—always right!

This adage should be your guiding light, for it marks a tectonic shift in the way leaders and managers in the industry must view their most significant stakeholder: the empowered **consumer**, not the disempowered **patient**.

Over the next few years, we will see a dramatic shift in the way healthcare is considered, promoted, configured, and purchased. We will hear extensive debate on the merits of this new approach, and whether it will really come to fruition, or if it's just a passing fad.

Much as we've seen in the financial sector with employee pensions (migrating from defined benefit to defined contribution), this is a movement whose time has come and whose impact is enormous.

Avoiding the fiscal fallout

Those who debate the merits of a consumer-centric plan but do not act will not only miss the movement but will be left in the proverbial dust, trying to apply yesterday's model to tomorrow's reality. Unfortunately, those who debate the merits of a consumer-oriented approach may include a significant number of individuals and enterprises, but the size of that group will not mitigate the immensity of their miscalculation or the competitively disadvantaged state in which they will find themselves.

Let's look at the factors that support the move to an optimized SL model.

Micro, not macro

Health executives may be tempted to believe that these seismic shifts could best be addressed at the full organizational level. However, logic dictates that to the extent that an organization is divided effectively into market-focused segments, major transitions are actually better assessed and accomplished under an optimized SL structure.

In essence, the rise of the healthcare consumer could also be aptly labeled "the emergence of the individual." SLM gets the enterprise closer to the individual than any other managerial model, which is why it is the mainstay of competitive consumer-oriented industries and organizations throughout the United States. Just ask the leaders at consumer goods firms, organizations known for their acumen in

SLM (or what they term product or product line management) how far they will go to know their customers' needs intimately.

And the focus on intimated consumer knowledge has only accelerated with the advent of the Internet. Savvy consumer-focused firms from Amazon to Starbucks have nearly perfected the art/science of individual interests and buying behavior with sophisticated real-time tracking mechanisms, predictive models, and economic behavior algorithms.

Although these may be different industries, the same reasoning holds true for healthcare: An organizational model that more closely aligns the operating units with the customer base is more strategically positioned to adapt to major market changes.

The need for flexibility

The current configuration of many hospitals does not allow for the market flexibility required by insurance exchanges and the implementation of the ACA, with a push for accountable care and population health. For comparison, consider why so many facilities suffered financially following the first few years of diagnosis-related group (DRG) implementation back in the mid-eighties, as well as the difficulty that enterprises had adjusting to the Balanced Budget Act (BBA) of 1997. The financial, operational, and accountability structure of most hospitals simply does not allow for timely and successful adaptation of a new delivery overlay.

It is clear that our healthcare system (including its hospitals and health systems) does not adjust well to sweeping change. Industry observers have noted that healthcare systems (and, to a lesser extent, hospitals) are about as maneuverable as supertankers. When faced with the need to change course—as a result of external forces or internal considerations—it takes extensive time and considerable effort to do so. This is understandable; however, it is not sustainable.

Responding to a competitive market

SLM enables an organization to assess its vulnerable areas rapidly and make necessary adjustments. It forces the organization to institute a discipline of measurement and accountability that exists in nearly every other industrial sector of American enterprise. Yet some healthcare leaders have balked at the need for such a structure, arguing that hospitals and health systems aren't actually selling products or offering consumer-oriented services. Yet that model is one that is shifting as the consumer becomes more economically engaged and cognitively empowered, as noted in the Foreword, and, as the competition shifts to market-facing organizations (e.g., retail chains) that do understand consumers, since that is their world.

At its most rudimentary level, SLM is merely a subdividing of the organization into manageable, measurable, and accountable components. That ability will be more important in the near future than ever before.

In part, that's because we face an onslaught of new and notable competitors. And although SLM is not a silver bullet for the threat of emerging competition, its organizational structure can improve the ability of a hospital or health system to preempt competition, compete effectively against them, or pursue a middle ground of partnership with potential competitors in the market.

In fundamental terms, SLM provides the focus on the core services or areas that are most important to the hospital: It assigns distinct and direct accountability to an individual or individuals to monitor the dynamics of the market and ensures that the organization is optimally positioned to protect, defend, and expand in those areas that are mission critical.

Conclusion

In summary, this book is designed to outline the framework for SL execution in a rapidly shifting market. These fundamentals, while not necessarily rudimentary, also are not rocket science. The basic principles are an outgrowth of my experience with SLM over the course of 25 years in the healthcare field, with the benefit of having applied these tenets and tactics in the packaged goods industry prior to my migration to healthcare. Here at the cusp of the emergence of the consumer, these principles offer a more timely application than ever before in the history of the healthcare industry.

2

Welcome to Our
Brave New World

A Mind-Set to Match the Market

Not only are evolving reimbursement models challenging providers, but the
industry's economic underpinnings have begun the shift from a "wholesale"
to more of a "retail" orientation. This is nothing short of a sea change for the
healthcare industry, which has its roots in two fundamentally hierarchical models:
the medical model on the clinical side (diagnose then prescribe) and the military
model on the administrative side. Neither of these models is consumer-savvy nor
particularly consumer-friendly, since a consumer-driven model places the end
purchaser in the position of ultimate power.

Few people would argue that healthcare has that kind of dynamic. Yet, as the
industry shifts to a retail model, and during a time when social networks have
emerged in every sector, the old hierarchical managerial models are under siege,
or soon will be, and the torch is being passed to the engaged and empowered
consumer.

Adding to the fun, a new wave of competition has emerged as a serious force in industry dynamics: Primary care providers and physician practices, hospital ERs, and even urgent-care centers all face the serious threat of big-box retailers like Walmart capturing a good share of their volume. When the largest retailer in the world wades into your territory, you know you're not going to have a positive outcome. And physicians, as well as the hospitals and health systems that support or employ them, face an increasing threat from Internet-based competitors like ZocDoc and iTriage.

Healthcare executives need more than new models to vanquish these threats. In truth, we need to adopt a new mind-set and, in so doing, adapt to this brave new world. The post–Affordable Care Act (ACA) world requires a number of shifts in managerial thinking in the healthcare setting.

1. Think of yourself as the CEO of your service line

In a post-ACA service line (SL) model, the SL director acting as a mini-CEO will maintain constant awareness of changing market conditions and emerging competition. Applying a CEO mentality to management, this director will be acutely aware of how to match resources to the demands of the individual consumer as well as to the collective populations required under an accountable care model. In reality, SL directors or vice presidents should function as mini-CEOs anyway, since they are in control of the destiny of their SLs. It's that kind of sense of urgency and ownership mentality that often separates the highly successful SL leaders from the average group.

During these times of unprecedented transition, if you adopt a CEO mind-set, you will develop and execute on an SL strategy optimized for the post-ACA world.

2. Develop a love for data analytics

Simply put, superior data management skills will separate the winners from the soon-to-be has-beens. And while any number of healthcare executives may consider themselves to be data driven, our current models are a far stretch from the sophistication of data analytics that will be required going forward. As will be discussed in greater depth in subsequent chapters, a data-driven approach and a deep understanding of and appreciation for analytics will be essential in a consumer-oriented environment, just as they currently are in leading market-driven industries and companies. There's a reason you can't read very far in any business publication without encountering the term "big data." Big data is more than the latest rage, it's the great differentiator.

3. Patients aren't traditional "patients" in a population health model

Your SLs must be optimized not simply to treat *disease* (i.e., sick care) but for a much more efficient, holistic, and humanistic model that focuses on keeping people healthy (i.e., true healthcare). When you develop a population health mind-set, your organization will benefit greatly, because it will make the shift from delivering episodic care to managing the health of a defined population. As obvious as that statement may seem, few organizations understand the fundamental premise of designing for a population health model or know how to prepare for and execute on that transition.

Obviously, the government has set the course with initiatives like Triple Aim, bundled payments, accountable care organizations, and so forth. And when the federal government—which pays an unconscionable amount of money into the healthcare coffers—decides to flex its considerable muscle, the system *will* change.

Making a commitment to adopt this new operating model and adapt your SLs to address population health will directly contribute to the long-term success of your organization. You will deliver quality care to consumers, earn their loyalty, and (not incidentally) position your organization for a successful adjustment to the revised payment schedules and models for reimbursement.

4. Consumers (millions of them) will be calling the shots

The next concept to bear in mind as you analyze your current SL strategy is the dramatic escalation of consumer involvement in health insurance and healthcare purchasing decisions. If you are to remain relevant and competitive in the market, you must understand what consumers expect, want, and need.

On the public side of the equation, health insurance exchanges—the cornerstone of the ACA—even with their troubled start have enrolled and empowered millions of individuals who heretofore had little or no insurance. This increasingly wide swath of the population will have a dramatic impact on the way healthcare is perceived, accessed, and delivered. And the emergence of this powerful new group has happened in a relatively brief time frame.

The migration to private health exchanges

In early September 2013, IBM announced that it was migrating most of its retirees (upward of 110,000) to a private exchange called Extend Health. At the time that announcement was made, Extend Health, which is headquartered in San Mateo, CA and is a division of Towers Watson, already had more than a half million enrollees. On the heels of the IBM decision, Time Warner announced that it too would move its retirees to an exchange model. One week after those significant announcements, Walgreens (officially known as The Walgreen Company), the largest drug retailing chain in the United States, announced that it was moving 120,000 of its employees to a private insurance exchange.

A number of other large retailers and manufacturers have followed suit, a trend that is likely to accelerate over the next few years. This significant movement among large, medium, and small employers amounts to a migration away from "defined benefit" toward a "defined contribution" model. Some industry experts see it as the beginning of the end for employer-sponsored health insurance. In the months and years ahead, we will likely see the majority of employers migrating their employees and retirees to either public or private exchanges.

It's very important to keep in mind that public health insurance exchanges are not the only force driving the framework of consumer engagement. Private health exchanges are also emerging as a viable force in the healthcare industry (see box).

Do not underestimate the impact that insurance exchanges will have on your SL strategy. With increased financial investment, consumers will become more personally invested, and the entire nature of the purchasing construct and delivery model will be dramatically altered.

5. Provide value; the money will follow

Expect that consumers participating in exchanges will question the *value* of the services they receive. These enrollees will purchase insurance as individuals and will make decisions based on personal needs. No longer will they pay, as so many have done historically, just a fraction of the total cost of their treatments and healthcare services.

You can expect the same focus on value from consumers whose employers do provide insurance (a number that has dropped precipitously over the past three decades) but are passing along much more of the financial responsibility to their employees.

Exchanges provide a direct tie between services rendered and fiscal accountability of the person who received them. That is called market orientation, and exchanges will drive consumers toward it.

6. Evolve

Organizational leaders must face the reality that the new world of healthcare will bear little resemblance to the one in which they have operated for decades. We can be fairly certain that the current *modus operandi* will not be the *modus operandi* for much longer.

What remains to be seen is whether executives and managers who have done well in the established model will successfully transition to a consumer-driven landscape, operating under a population health overlay.

7. Focus on cost control AND profit enhancement

Profit margins won't be diminished in relation to effective cost control; in fact, margins should be enhanced. Under a robust SL structure, the organization will strategically target its cost-cutting efforts in a way that aligns the enterprise resources with market needs and consumer demands.

This point deserves considerable emphasis. The current approach of too many healthcare systems and hospitals is to implement across-the-board cuts when money is tight and belts need tightening. This approach is both suboptimal and arguably ineffective: Across-the-board reductions and wholesale cost cutting are often reactive and typically fail to retain the resources (i.e., people, programs, and promotion) of those services that are contributing the most to the overall benefit of the organization. A sophisticated SL structure and execution takes a much more strategic approach to rightsizing and therefore positions the organization more effectively and symmetrically within the market in which it operates.

8. Fear not

Progressive leaders will emerge and make this transition effectively and successfully. Realize that the world is changing, so the senior leadership team must change with it or face the consequences of being competitively outmaneuvered.

Don't maintain the status quo by offering outdated models and pursuing old strategies with outmoded approaches. Fear of change can be paralyzing, but it obviously will not be the operating approach of progressive leaders; effective, progressive leaders embrace change as the new normal. They not only welcome the challenge of adapting to a new environment and adopting a new *modus operandi*, but they also enjoy the turbulent time of transition and the rush of navigating uncharted waters.

9. To get close to your customers, get close to your physicians

Work closely with physicians and clinicians to move toward a data-driven approach, both at the individual patient level and in the aggregate when managing the care of a defined population.

Savvy SL directors and managers now understand what some of us have been advocating for years—namely, that for SLs to move beyond a mere organizational construct (with the requisite meetings, business plans, and promotional campaigns), key physicians within those SLs must be integrated into the model, the plan development, and the strategy execution.

The coleader organization design, one that includes physician leaders as integral to the structure, provides a management model that is consistent with the times. In addition to ensuring buy-in from key members and leaders of the medical staff (and, through the trickle-down effect, most medical staff members), it enhances loyalty among the medical staff. Substantive engagement may even discourage competitive ventures by members of the medical staff. And that is no small feat.

One case in point is a health system in Boise, Idaho, that effectively incorporated a structure of physician coleaders in its SL model. Each service line is managed by the SL director and a physician coleader, who provides invaluable insight and perspective from the medical viewpoint. Of course, in many of the nation's leading systems that are cited for their integration and coordination (such as The Cleveland Clinic, Mayo Clinic, Intermountain Health Care, or Geisinger), this type of physician-centered structure is inherent in the very operating model.

Because members of the medical staff are often the greatest source of competition for hospitals and health systems, employing a collaboration-promoting structure has great intrinsic value, and, as noted above, it will be essential to success under a population health construct.

Forays on the frontier

One fine example of a shift to physician co leadership can be seen in northwest Montana, where the executives at Kalispell Regional Medical Center (KRMC) applied a model of SL development that involved the entire community and key stakeholders, from the board of directors to the foundation.

The community was in great need of a breast cancer specialist following the announcement that the venerable physician who had devoted much of his professional practice to treating women with breast disease was retiring. In successfully filling that void, the leadership team at KRMC enlisted a core group of patients of this particular physician in educating and galvanizing key community leaders. An effort was launched to recruit a highly trained and board-certified specialist in the area of breast oncologic surgery and, to do so, to make a commitment to building an entire Center for Breast Health.

The energy, enthusiasm, and sheer momentum of the movement became so compelling and convincing that a major donor in Texas offered to fund the center's development and provided more than $1 million in funding. A key physician was identified, and leaders of the community, including board members, many members of the medical staff, and the breast cancer survivors' interest group, hosted a reception to introduce the physician to the community and to the opportunity.

Even though this highly trained physician had offers to practice in some of the most prestigious centers in the country, and in much larger metropolitan settings, she chose Kalispell (a community of fewer than 40,000 people) in large part due to the commitment to the model and the general enthusiasm for and interest in her area of expertise.

Interestingly, not long after the program opened, the recruited physician was able to identify that the breast cancer screening rate was low in the catchment area, particularly in a number of the smaller communities that lacked services. Responding to this community need, KRMC purchased and operated a mobile mammography unit or what they call a "coach." The mobile mammography unit travels throughout Northwestern Montana and offers services in conjunction with critical access hospitals, helping to eliminate traditional barriers to care by making the screening process faster and more convenient for women in the rural areas of the state. The same group that organized to bring the initial endeavor to fruition continues to offer support to the overall effort by periodically holding fundraising events, the proceeds of which provide financial assistance to those individuals unable to pay for the screenings. Jane Winkley, a local resident, philanthropist, and breast cancer survivor and the woman for whom the KRMC Winkley Women's Center was named, provided the funding for the mobile coach.

All of this speaks to the extensive community benefit that an SL can provide if the leaders within the hospital or health system effectively galvanize key stakeholders and all those for which the SL offers inherent value.

10. Coordinated care = continuum of care

Coordination is what the consumer expects and requires. In the summer of 2013, this point was empirically validated in an extensive consumer research study by BVK, a well-known healthcare ad agency in Milwaukee. In this consumer preference study, BVK surveyed more than 1,500 consumers regarding their awareness of healthcare trends, terms, and interests.

Interestingly, when the survey respondents were asked about their awareness and opinion of "accountable care," they were both unaware and uninterested in that terminology. Rather, what these representative consumers said was "most important" to them was "coordinated" care, and they felt that systems that would earn their business would offer that critical element of healthcare delivery.

This type of inclusive involvement by several parties may not work for all SLs or in many health systems or hospitals, but the creativity is worthy of note and of merit. The key takeaway from this and other inventive applications is the need to adjust the application to the needs of the patients/consumers within the market and to involve key stakeholders in the process.

An SL structure allows the organizational model to do just that, as well as to provide so many other underpinnings necessary to achieving market success in these demanding yet opportunistic times.

Conclusion

Too many times in the business setting, whether manufacturing, retail, or healthcare, the main focus is on the operating model. Certainly, there is incredible value and empirical success in adopting a model that aligns with the shifting demands of the market. However, what is sometimes overlooked or undervalued, particularly in times of dramatic change, is the need for a new managerial mind-set to choreograph that transition.

This is particularly true in the healthcare field, especially in the provider sector, where the operating model has experienced only nominal change over the past few decades. Yet, to adapt to the kind of change we expect and, in fact, are now experiencing as a result of the move to population health and the emergence of the empowered healthcare consumer, nothing short of a modified mind-set among leaders will be essential to long-term success. Few would argue that the healthcare field is in the throes of unprecedented change, yet how many leaders have recognized the need to revisit and revise their basic worldview of the industry or their managerial mind-set?

The first step in envisioning and then embracing that new mind-set is to understand how market dynamics will change and then to adopt an organizational structure that aligns with that altered landscape. Based on the experience of a number of industries and thousands of companies, the SL structure is a proven framework for sensing the shifts in the market and staying close to the consumer/patient.

3

Why Exchanges Change Everything

Much has been written about the advent of the health insurance exchange (HIX), the politically charged cornerstone of the Affordable Care Act (ACA), but not enough consideration has been given to its sweeping impact on our industry, from both a market dynamic perspective, and as a fundamental shift in control, with the consumer/patient emerging in a much more central role than ever before. This change will have major ramifications for the entire healthcare system.

System, Health Thyself

For decades, the reimbursement for the major share of U.S. healthcare provided to the private sector has been supported by the architecture of the employer-sponsored insurance (ESI) model, a construct that noted health industry writer Paul Starr referred to as a "recipe for disaster" due to the fact that the end user is not the principal purchaser.

Some claim that the patient's detachment from economic responsibility drives the disproportionately lower value (i.e., outcomes compared to costs) in U.S. health services relative to every other industrialized nation in the world; however, that detachment is about to change.

With the advent of healthcare exchanges, individual purchasers of care will soon be intimately involved in the finances of healthcare. End users are about to develop a vested interest in the quality of care through the investment of their hard-earned dollars. And as that seismic shift occurs, all healthcare organizations—especially providers—will need to take proactive steps to meet the challenges of this new initiative.

Steady-State No Longer

The healthcare industry and its basic "minimal outlay for services rendered" equation has remained relatively unchanged over the past four decades. Admittedly, there have been major changes in the reimbursement structure and payment architecture with the advent of Medicare and Medicaid in the mid-sixties, and the introduction of diagnosis-related groups in the mid-eighties. There have also been some significant disruptive forces in the payment structure with the introduction of health maintenance organizations (HMO) and other insurance-related models and vehicles.

But despite these changes, the basic "exchange" dynamic between consumer/patient and provider has remained virtually the same. Even with the rise of HMOs, consumers were never really empowered to take control of their care or to manage their own health; in fact, HMOs left Jill and Joe Consumer/Patient feeling less empowered and more frustrated by the lack of choice in providers, namely physicians and hospitals that they could select.

In the past decade, however, consumer and patients have started to shoulder a larger segment of the overall cost burden for healthcare/medical services. Slowly but steadily, employers have started to share the cost with their employees, increasing the amount of copays, deductibles, and percent of premium that employees must pony up. And while this has not gone without notice (or without a certain element of employee disgruntlement), most are willing to absorb this added cost.

Why? Likely because many are simply grateful that their employer still offers insurance at all and is still picking up the lion's share of the tab. Even though most mid- to large-size employers still offer healthcare insurance for their employees, the ranks of those covered by ESI have dwindled considerably over the past two decades, from more than 80% in 1980 to just less than 60% in 2010. Understandably, then, employers have some leverage when they ask or require their employees to shoulder an increasing share of the cost burden.

Precedent and Proof of a Market Already in Motion

The introduction of health insurance exchanges marks the beginning of the end for third-party financial accountability and the onset of true consumerism in healthcare. Insurance exchanges (or marketplaces) precipitated two note-worthy changes: They have accelerated the march toward increased financial accountability for the consumer/patient, and they opened the door for employers to offer an alternative to the ESI model.

The fact is that employers don't necessarily want to provide insurance as it's currently configured. In a moment of total candor, many HR executives will admit that in its current form, insuring employees is a hassle in terms of the time and resources it takes, and the distraction from core operating business. Many firms would readily exit the business altogether if they could ... and if their competitors were willing to do the same. The implementation of exchanges opens that door gradually by introducing the option for individuals and small employers—followed by the mid-size and eventually large employers—to provide a set amount of dollars for health insurance to their employees. Under this new arrangement/model, the individual employee can deal with the "fun" of navigating the health system, while the employer virtually exits the game altogether and focuses on its fundamental reason for being.

I'm not the first to predict that this exodus of employers will happen over the next several years, but I do think it will happen more rapidly than most have postulated. And just what evidence do we have to support that prediction, you ask? At least two historical precedents.

HMOs

The first precedent, the significant emergence of HMOs, occurred in the late eighties and early nineties. The concept of capitated care under an HMO had been around since the early seventies, when, during the Nixon Administration, it was signed into law. Still, HMOs kind of hobbled along and never got much traction until the mid-eighties, when a few large employers decided they would try the model to reduce costs. It soon spread like wildfire, and HMO penetration went from less than 5% in the early to mid-eighties to nearly 50% of all insured employees just a decade later.

We've learned from that experience and others that once a major player in a particular industry takes the plunge, competitors soon follow. A few pundits have suggested that, of the large firms, the telecommunications industry may be the first to take that leap when it comes to insurance exchanges. If that prediction does prove true, once that segment of American industry makes the migration to exchanges (public or private), other large companies and entire industries will follow. As we've seen, large and storied companies such as IBM, Time Warner, and Walgreens have led the way by transferring either their retirees or their actual employees to private exchanges.

Pension funding

The second precedent was the seismic shift that occurred in how pensions were funded throughout most of the nation and with most employers.

Not all that long ago, many employers (especially large enterprises) provided their employees with a pension based on defined benefit (i.e., an established amount), sometimes pegged to inflation over the course of a retiree's life after leaving the firm. As we've observed, that model has pretty much gone the way of video stores and cassette tapes.

Very few firms or even public entities continue to offer defined benefit plans, owing to the considerable fiscal liability they face with retiree benefit packages. Instead, most employers have shifted to defined contribution plans, wherein they encourage their employees to save for retirement in 401(k) or 403(b) plans. As an incentive, many employers provide matching contributions.

So what does that have to do with health insurance and the move toward individual accountability? Health insurance could be viewed as the "second-wave-cousin" of pension plans. Over time, employers will likely migrate their employees to insurance products that resemble 401(k) plans for retirement. These arrangements give the employees more control over their health insurance decisions and more accountability for the expenditure of their money—even if the funds are provided by the employer. Importantly, from the employer's vantage, the increase in health-related contribution accounts can be pegged to a more predictable index (like inflation or general cost of living) and not to the stratospherically volatile indices like medical costs and insurance premiums, which have consistently outpaced standard inflation measures by an annual factor of three to four times throughout the decade.

What's not to like about that arrangement from the employer's standpoint? In actuality, very little, especially if competitors pursue the same strategy.

Exchanges and the Digital Connection

If the rise of the Internet produced the democratization of American healthcare, then exchanges are likely to produce the digital empowerment of the healthcare consumer and the final digital coming-of-age for the industry. Although the Internet has already provided valuable inroads into a seemingly impenetrable field (from an accessibility to information standpoint), the nascent nature of real consumerism in healthcare has no doubt held the full force of the digital conversion at bay.

Consequently, the data analytics that apply to healthcare derive historically and largely from a clinical quality perspective, not from a consumer-centric standpoint. For example, the consumer-oriented databases and applications that companies like Amazon, Starbucks, Apple, and Marriott gather and utilize are not even on the radar for many healthcare organizations. When healthcare executives or consultants talk about the use of "big data" and sophisticated data analytics, as with the "Moneyball" model (from the film based on the life of the Oakland A's general manager, Billy Beane), it is not necessarily with the consumer in mind.

In this regard, the insurance companies have a distinct advantage over the provider sector in that they have vast reservoirs of data regarding the members in their plans, how they use health services, and their general behavioral patterns when it comes to the purchase of healthcare. However, even the large insurance companies have not mined the mountains of consumer data on which they sit to the extent they could or should. Much of that is changing, as indicated by the largest insurance companies who have purchased sophisticated data management enterprises that specialize in the art and science of transforming reams of data into accurately and intimately applied consumer intelligence. These firms effectively apply the data, using purchaser behavioral algorithms, to focus on behavioral economics in the way that leading data-centric, consumer-facing firms like those mentioned earlier have done for years.

This type of analysis is relatively new to most of the health industry and certainly virgin territory for the provider sector. Yet, that is about to change with the convergence of consumerism, the move toward population health, and a shift in the basic reimbursement model from episodic care to the management of a defined population over time. With consumers economically "on the hook" and providers soon to be responsible for managing the health of defined populations, this industry is about to join its more advanced colleagues in commerce. When that day arrives, the power of the digital movement will be unleashed, and the entire dynamic of communicating to, connecting with, and being continuously assessed by the vocal masses will rock this industry to its core.

As digital experts like to say, networks eventually override hierarchies. If ever there was an industry that remains locked in its historically hierarchical ways, it is healthcare, at least those on the traditional delivery side of the fence. Consequently, the emergence of digitization and the sweeping power of networks (which always follows that kind of consumer-driven digitization coup) will be quite a sight to see and quite a challenge for organizations that hold on to yesterday's model.

Progressive organizations and the far-sighted leaders that run them don't have to be overrun by the technological tsunami. Rather, they can choose to ride the wave and stay above it. One of the best ways to do that is through a service line (SL) structure, with the SL manager/director serving as a key convener and responder to the networks that emerge.

Conclusion

The introduction of exchanges can be viewed as the proverbial match that ignites an imminent wild fire. Not only will the general industry construct move from a wholesale model to a retail model, but consumers will demand the kind of information, accessibility, and convenience that they require and demand from other industries. Since it will be their money on the line, they will be more engaged as active participants and decision-makers. That emerging market dynamic is both exciting and daunting. And that is one reason why SL architecture is so vital to a successful strategy under the new insurance exchange environment.

Product line/SLM has been tried and tested in virtually every other industry in the nation, and it keeps emerging as the optimal structure for getting closer (and staying closer) to the consumer. The healthcare industry, in this era of transition and transformation, is no different than the rest.

4

Service Line Applications to Population Health

Service line management (SLM) has been part of the healthcare industry for more than three decades, but for some reason, the model hasn't been applied nearly as effectively as it could have and should have been. In the near future, however, SLM will experience both a renaissance and a heightened appreciation for the value it offers progressive hospitals and health systems.

Like newly discovered talent on a reality TV show, SL strategy is poised to experience a dramatic increase in popularity among healthcare executives. As noted earlier, much of the appreciation for well-crafted and high-performing SLs will result from their close alignment with more fiscally involved consumers in the healthcare sector.

This chapter explores the other chief market dynamic that will escalate the adoption of refined SL constructs: the healthcare industry's unfaltering march toward population health. Population health initiatives that result from an optimized SL model will offer strategic solutions tailored to key populations.

To that end, let's review the options and the tools available to execute on your consumer alignment strategies.

Aligning Your SL with Population Health

Why would optimizing your SL strategy for population health produce even more benefits than a consumer focus alone? The answer to that question deserves several pages on its own, but it can be attributed to two key realities:

- First, population health is already prominently displayed on the radar screen of the big three functional areas in healthcare: clinicians, operators, and financial types. In essence, this is one of the highest if not the highest priority for executives and managers in each of these areas.

- Second, population health is much more familiar territory than consumer alignment. The health industry attempted (and largely failed) to embrace a population health mind-set with the managed care movement and the drive toward integrated delivery systems in the nineties. Even though that initial foray failed, this second-stage iteration has the backing of the federal government, as well as the interest and infrastructure of key stakeholders throughout the industry. Consequently, most people think it will actually stick this time.

What many don't yet understand is that SLs offer one of the most effective avenues for capturing patient/consumer "capitated" payments, as well as for managing the health of defined populations. Well-designed and effectively managed SLs have the potential to offer comprehensive solutions for each subsegment of a defined population, particularly those individuals who utilize healthcare services the most and who therefore account for the lion's share of the resources expended.

For population health to be truly effective, the full continuum of care needs to be efficiently coordinated, including unprecedented interaction with both consumer and patient. I purposefully make this distinction at this point because in the future consumer interactions will very likely be as important as those involving the patient. The emphasis will be on working with and caring for individuals prior to their needing treatment and the provision of healthcare services. The very nature of the reimbursement architecture will drive this new interactive model.

Why? Because the full network that is attending to the defined population (including the healthy and the not-so-healthy) will need to reach out to individuals and families well in advance of their requiring healthcare. With a population health orientation, the network of providers—hospitals, clinics, physicians, nurses, post-acute clinicians, and so forth—will have an interest in identifying and monitoring the individuals who need education, information, and self-directed care well before they begin utilizing the services.

Consequently, successful healthcare organizations will provide a continuum of services that will deliver the appropriate education, health regimen, preventive services, and (as somewhat of a "last resort") diagnosis and treatment for those members within the population who require traditional acute care services. This is particularly true for the segment of the defined population that utilizes 80% (or higher) of the resources available.

Data, Data Everywhere

This high-profile, high-wire balancing act of population health management is an ideal framework for big data. Yet amassing and reviewing data for data's sake is not the answer. Much of the data that is being packaged right now won't provide the insight needed to effectively manage a defined population, because it represents an impressive array of extensive but often tangential **statistics**.

The data management and monitoring approach that will achieve meaningful empirical results for accountable care organizations will focus on individual patterns, characteristics, and behavior. Data configuration and utilization must emphasize understanding, monitoring, and, where necessary, changing behavior in a way that is beneficial for the individual and for the overall system.

Thanks to the digital tracking and sophisticated analytic models, we have learned from observing other industries that consumer behavior is fundamentally quite predictable. We've also seen that most consumers don't mind the individualized attention and the specifically tailored product and service applications that result from the use of behavioral science. In healthcare, we have only begun to scratch the surface with the type of digitally driven, individual-specific models that will benefit society and improve our health, but we expect to see similar outcomes.

We have arrived at the intersection of consumerism and population health; and this is where SL strategy may yet prove its highest worth. Case in point, of all the staff in a healthcare organization, the market-facing employees, including marketers and SL managers, are arguably the most adept at using a consumer-facing model because they are already comfortable with and responsible for interacting with the consumer, as well as with the patient.

Consumer-Facing Applications by Market-Facing Professionals

Given that some organizations are already employing advanced versions of an SL approach, how can healthcare organizations apply the SL model more effectively for population health?

Customer relationship management (CRM) has begun to morph into a **customer enterprise model (CEM).** This transformation (which is already underway in some hospitals) follows what we're seeing in other industries, in particular within the technology field. Under this model, the customer becomes the enterprise to which the organization is marketing. Technologies such as the iPhone have turned the entire exchange relationship pyramid upside down, placing the customer at the center of the market universe. Healthcare will eventually adapt to this model (call it iHealth) as the patient becomes the enterprise, drawing individualized attention. The organizations that lead this charge will be progressive enterprises that are attuned to the needs of the market and the desires of the individual.

Psychographic mapping and **targeted messaging** are two more ways that healthcare organizations can more effectively apply the SL model. Healthcare organizations have not fully adopted these accepted techniques for applying

30

precision messages and individualized services or customized products, but the number of hospitals and health systems that are using them is increasing. This trend goes hand in hand with CEM, yet it often precedes the tailored restructuring of the organization's offerings in the market. Psychographic mapping and targeted messaging have been used in multiple industries with great success, but it is only now gaining traction in healthcare as consumers exercise more clout and demand more directed communication.

Some sophisticated organizations are applying targeted messaging in a **specificity to disease** approach. What this means in terms of SLM is drilling down into the diagnosis-related group (DRG), ICD-9/ICD-10, or ambulatory payment classification (APC) level to fine-tune incremental marketing efforts.

Figure 4.1 | Psychographic mapping vs. traditional (demographic) mapping

Demographic Mapping	Psychographic Mapping
Income	Purchasing behavior
Education	Personal interests
Age	Technology acumen
Gender	Hobbies
Ethnicity	Cultural factors

A few organizations are able to utilize fairly sophisticated software applications to segment patient population by payer-code category. One typical approach is to slice patient data to look at all the patients treated for a particular event, such as "major chest procedures, surgical" (MSDRG 168). Marketers and SL managers then profile this segment of the patient universe by demographic, sociographic, and some elements of psychographic data. Then, via a combination of ZIP code and Web-based outreach, they are able to target the appropriate marketing messages and information to this market segment.

The MSDRG 168 payer-code subsegment produces a higher margin, so it merits allocation of increased resources for the objective of realizing new business. Using this rather standard approach, a hospital or health system can target a specific message to attract incremental patients for that particular treatment and that specific market segment.

Admittedly, some leaders in the industry might bristle at this level of targeted messaging and market segmentation, arguing that it runs counter to a mission of treating all the people in the community. Remember, however, that this type of segmentation does not mean that the hospital is denying care to any population, or even restricting its care to an "elite" slice of the community. Rather, this is a situation where the hospital is focusing on higher-margin incremental patient volume. Successful hospitals and health systems realize that they must balance the wide-swath population portfolio with incremental growth that provides more favorable reimbursement. This strategy provides a way to offset the vast number of patients in payer classes/categories that reimburse below the cost of providing the services. It's the business model application of the oft-cited reality of "No margin, no mission." This is particularly true for nonprofit facilities that often see a disproportionate share of self-pay, Medicaid, Medicare, and charity care patients.

Furthermore, including a targeted segmentation strategy makes perfect sense in a market environment where organizations are struggling to stay afloat, given the increasing level of bad debt and declining reimbursement from government payers. In essence, targeted segmentation embodies a higher-margin, center-of-excellence focus, in which SLs that offer more favorable reimbursement due to the mix of procedural services (such as cardiology, neuroscience, or orthopedics) support the lower-margin lines of the hospital.

This approach can be applied to any and every SL, isolating the sub segments of each SL population to focus on higher-margin segments. Targeted segmentation is a mainstay of SLM, and it is the main reason that the model has been so effective in other industries.

Note from the field

When we first developed the SL model for Sacred Heart Hospital in Eugene, Oregon, more than 25 years ago, the differentiating feature of our approach was this very element highlighted above—namely, a drill-down on each SL population. Due to the unsophisticated nature of data availability and configuration at that time, the assessment mechanism was designed to determine margin prioritization and review options for improving efficiency, revamping coding practices, or even "de-marketing" a particular subsegment of the SL (in some cases, this resulted in scaling back on the promotion and development of particular services or treatments due to unfavorable reimbursement).

In today's world of sophisticated software packages that can not only array the data by individual payer code and treatment category but also provide vast amounts of background information on each patient, the possibilities for true market segmentation and tailored messaging more closely parallel the models utilized in best-practice consumer or manufacturing industries. However, in both applications—that of 25 years past as well as today—the heart of the approach is an emphasis on data.

Even very advanced organizations—those that are taking SLM to the next level and mimicking what occurs in savvy sectors of American industry—begin with the definitional aspects of SLM. They use commercial software applications that provide mountains of data on the core SLs as well as SL subsegments.

Shifting the Pricing Paradigm

Healthcare marketing is atypical from other industry applications in many ways, but in the pricing realm, it is a definite anomaly.

As any marketing student or practitioner will attest, pricing is one of the fundamentals under the purview of marketing (one of the "four Ps" to use Phillip Kotler's timeless terminology). Yet in the healthcare sector, pricing is not only coordinated and controlled by another function (usually managed care or finance), but marketing is rarely involved in basic service pricing configuration or in discussions about pricing models and applications. Arguably, the primary reason for this divergence from accepted marketing practices of other industries is the heretofore disengaged and "unempowered" consumer.

Consumers/patients are now taking a more active role. Leading systems recognize both the emerging trends and current opportunities, and they utilize the SL forum to pursue more retail-oriented, market-based pricing. For example, some systems use highly sophisticated software algorithms (the same used for the airline industry) to differentiate "commodity services" (i.e., those available in every hospital or ambulatory setting) from "proprietary services" (i.e., those available in tertiary or quaternary facilities). With this type of differentiated pricing, it is possible for a hospital to renegotiate its rates with payers and become much more competitive with emerging players, such as physician-owned entities or entrepreneurial ventures.

In fact, one major hospital system in the Southwest used this pricing technique so effectively that the organization experienced a *downturn* in volumes—but a significant increase in net revenue and operating margins—as a function of strategic and differentiated pricing. That is very much on the horizon for savvy leaders with an SL mentality: the type of customized pricing ability that will tailor the pricing of a particular service to the needs of the individualized patient.

As the nation moves away from an employer-based health insurance model and toward the individualized financing model, an optimized SL approach with subservice segmentation capabilities and a more tailored delivery model will offer a distinct competitive differentiation.

Progressive health leaders also recognize the need to have a market-oriented pricing model that provides both greater transparency for the consumer and a more competitive price structure in general. Many hospital and health system executives are in denial that the day will come when prices for their services are as available to the public as those of airlines and hotels, but that day is probably not more than three to four years out.

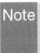 The current trend toward medical tourism (i.e., high-end services available in other nations at a fraction of the cost) is a harbinger of the customized pricing that we will see in advanced markets in the next five to 10 years.

The optimal framework for crafting patient-customized, market-savvy pricing is the same one that exists in other industries: an SL configuration.

Move Away from Affirmative Market Research

The healthcare industry (at least the provider sector) seems to be somewhat allergic to significant use of market research. Most of what is termed "research" conducted by hospitals and health systems focuses on patient, physician, and/or employee satisfaction surveys.

While these surveys do have their place and their role, they've traditionally been used to **affirm** rather than **inform**—that is, they provided *affirmation* that the current approach was working rather than *information* on the necessary operational and process changes that would lead to substantive change. In more recent years, with the second wave of the quality movement and its emphasis on everything from Six Sigma to the Six Pillars, there has been a heightened focus on actually correlating various stakeholders' experiences to quality improvement and perception.

These efforts are to be applauded, as they have moved the needle for many organizations (witness the number of hospitals or health systems that have won the Malcolm Baldridge Award) and have been applied and accelerated by the still-emerging pay-for-performance movement. Yet these satisfaction surveys most often focus on current business, namely today's customers, rather than on how the organization can anticipate and meet the needs of tomorrow's patients. In essence, market research, as it is currently configured and conducted, is mostly about delivering on yesterday's model, not about anticipating tomorrow's market dynamic and the consumer's wants or needs.

Anticipating tomorrow's needs in this way is the role and responsibility of good consumer market research, particularly in light of a population health application *(indicator)*. Such research also offers insight into how the organization can anticipate future demands *(revelator)*.

From a predictive standpoint, consumer research (of the general public, not of patients) can be a good leading indicator of market share. Case in point, if a hospital has a share of 45% in its defined market, and its consumer research indicates that only 40% of the randomly selected participants prefer that hospital to its competitors, then the hospital can probably expect some share decline in the next few years.

The converse is also true: When the preference share exceeds the actual market share, the hospital can usually anticipate an increase in market share over the near term. There are—of course—many factors to consider when assessing this measure, but on the whole, competitor preference is a fairly strong and reliable leading indicator of market share expectation.

Progressive organizations will tap into competitor preference as a leading indicator at the SL level, and they will conduct their awareness, quality perception, and competitor preference research by SL. For example, if a hospital's cardiovascular services are preferred by 65% of the population and the hospital currently has a 75% share, then that SL is likely headed for a downturn, or a reduction in its share of the market.

In terms of SL preference and its direct alignment with regional market share, the timetable may be a bit longer than with overall organizational market share and the alignment with consumer preference. This variance is due to the number of patients involved at both levels, with an obviously larger number at the overall market share level. However, using the SL consumer preference to gauge market share is still a fairly reliable indicator. Consequently, organizations that want to assess their market position in relation to the competition should conduct the appropriate research frequently and monitor the trends for movement and requisite action.

Carefully designed and well-conducted consumer research will reveal emerging trends related to the individual SLs and their market competitors and should therefore provide valuable insight into where consumers/patients are likely to direct their loyalty and use of services. In essence, research provides a great bellwether for the organization, as well as for specific SLs.

The Big (box) Bang Theory

The rise of convenience care clinics offers one example of the revelatory nature of market research and its relevance to SLM. Started around 2002, the model did not take serious root until around 2004 or 2005, by which time organizations like "Minute Clinics" (one of the pioneering firms in that space) were gaining a foothold in many markets, and the model was being pursued by major retail outlets or pharmacy chains (for example, Minute Clinics was eventually purchased by the CVS Pharmacy chain).

By early 2007, the field was quite crowded, with Walmart announcing that it would stake a major presence in the space and incorporate several thousand in-store clinics within a few years. Walmart took it a step further in 2012 and announced that it intended to eventually be "the largest provider of primary care in America."

Even with all that market noise and obvious movement, most hospitals and health systems were noticeably late to the convenient care party and therefore had to play catch-up. Yet, if hospital executives had invested relatively little effort on market research in those earlier days of the emerging convenient care model, they would have ascertained what the forerunners had already realized: that the model is viable *and* valuable in consumers' minds and in their share of the wallet.

Market research and reconnaissance designed to produce important revelations relative to consumer/patient preference and purchasing behavior is best organized and conducted under the auspices of the SL framework. For example, the above-cited preference for convenient care services would have likely been recognized by a hospital or health system with a functioning SL model that was measuring and monitoring referral streams to specialists. In such an organization, the SL team would have rapidly mobilized to determine the potential impact of the convenience care threat on their referral stream, conducted research to assess the organization's most useful and strategic approach, and then presented findings and recommendations to the senior leadership of the hospital.

Such is the rapid-fire assessment, recommendation, and execution triple-play model required in today's shifting market, and it is optimally configured with an SL model.

Conclusion

SLM is unique in its ability to offer a tailored approach to key stakeholders, whether physicians, patients, or patient families. We are beginning to see hospitals and health systems strategically leveraging their SLs for population health outreach, with detailed patient profiles, targeted direct mailings that have customized psychographic algorithms as their basis, and programmed services that cater to the individualized preferences of the targeted population.

Progressive organizations are incorporating this type of customization into their electronic communication (e.g., Web-based scheduling, billing, connectivity to physician offices, etc.). They are providing sophisticated communication interface and information exchange with the various operational components of their entire enterprise. What has been available in other sectors of the customer economy (from banks to beverage businesses) is now, finally, making serious headway into the healthcare realm, which one senior executive at a major computer firm referred to as "the last bastion of information-exchange inefficiency in the nation."

Progress, however, is about more than just information exchange and online ability. The iHealth movement, which involves focused communication and individualized messaging, is perhaps the most transformational change in healthcare—and it's right around the corner. Organizations that refine and align their SL managerial models with this market-based maelstrom will achieve a competitive differentiation the likes of which we have rarely seen in this field.

5

The Basic Framework for Service Line Execution

As simplistic as it may sound, most organizations can achieve service line (SL) success by adopting and adhering to just a handful of rules. Over the nearly three decades of SL implementation in healthcare, hospitals or health systems that employed the fundamental principles we'll explore in this chapter have proven much more successful in reaping the benefits of the SL model.

Although the competitive ground seems to shift under our feet, these precepts and principles remain largely intact; they have been proven time after time in economic sectors outside healthcare. Importantly—and this is a point worth underscoring—the practice of an optimized SL strategy and structure will be even more effective than ever before as our industry moves into a realm of heightened consumer engagement.

In other words, there has never been a better time to go back to the basics. Organizations following these elemental ground rules will experience favorable results in a relatively short time. As a bonus, those organizations will position themselves more competitively within the market, against their competitors.

A Playbook for Performance

Based on my experience and empirical research, the following rules for executing an effective SL structure are designed to be followed sequentially, and you should view them that way, as they build on each other for optimal execution:

1. Define the basic structure of the SLs in a measurable/quantifiable fashion. Determine the appropriate criteria for profiling the SLs in a way that enables comparison both within the organization and within the overall market.

2. Determine what really matters to the organization; then measure it to assess success. Establish the basic quantitative (or qualitative) metrics that the organization references in its accountability to key stakeholders—including the board of directors, physicians, employers, the corporate parent, and others.

3. Narrow the number of lines down to a manageable few—no more than four and perhaps as few as two—in order to allocate resources and concentrate effort.

4. Establish the (optimal) organizational design for SLs, depending on factors such as existing competition, internal resources, enterprise objectives, and leadership and governance intent.

5. Evaluate the organization's market position by SL, or in essence, how the individual business units match up against those of the competition.

6. Develop a business plan for each SL that syncs with the strategic plan. Surprisingly, many organizations have not established a forum and format for individual SL business plans that both flow from and fold up into the enterprise's long-range plan. This is essential both to unify the SL team and to ensure accountability and organizational buy-in.

7. Compete strategically at the micromarket level (i.e., the customer or key stakeholder). One reason hospitals and health systems have lost so much ground to niche players and emerging competitors is they are competing at the wrong level. They are focused broadly, rather than narrowly and strategically at the exchange entity's level.

8. Update the SL plan and model periodically to reflect changes in the market. As with effective strategic planning at the broader organizational level, SL planning should be ongoing and fluid enough to adapt to market shifts and competitive considerations.

These ground rules provide the basic scaffolding for a successful SL execution. The inherent efficiency and effectiveness of your revamped SL application will come into focus as the organization progresses through these precepts.

> **Note** One challenge of SLM, and the reason for its failure in many organizations, is that it is difficult to understand and implement at the outset. I recommend employing a sequential, systematic approach as the best path to helping the organization derive its core business identifications (i.e., key SLs) and mission-critical strategies and success factors.

1. Define SLs in a Measurable/Quantifiable Fashion

Think of this ground rule as the foundation of your home. If the foundation is hastily designed or ill constructed, the entire edifice will likely be substandard.

SL definition is hard work, because this is the point at which politics, traditions, and territory can muddy the picture and derail the effort. The organization's leaders must take an objective and data-driven approach to ensure that each subsequent element can be followed. Definition is usually the most time-consuming and discussion-provoking part of the process. It's often extremely frustrating, as it seems like the momentum is slowing and the model will never see the light of day.

In application, the definition of SLs simply needs to be a decision by senior management. This can be accomplished via a traditional data-driven approach (which I have recommended for years), using established categories or disease classifications. Alternatively, the organization can choose to identify and manage SLs with a commercial enterprise approach, focusing on patients that are interested in all the services and offerings under a broad category, such as women's health. Finally, and more frequently in recent years, SLs can be defined as very specific applications or consumer-related service offerings, such as bariatric surgery, wellness services, or even complementary and alternative medicine services.

Some of these latter options will be explored later in the book, but for now, we'll press forward with my recommendations for the more traditional approaches for employing data in your SL definition process.

Using ICD or DRG categories for measurement

Many SL traditionalists and seasoned managers recommend using diagnosis-related groups (DRG) or the International Classification of Diseases (ICD) for the inpatient (IP), outpatient (OP), and ambulatory patient group measure. As virtually everyone in the industry knows, 2014 marked the ICD framework transition from ICD-9 to ICD-10. The new version is considerably more thorough and granular, which, understandably, will make SL definition by ICD categorization more complex. These are not the only criteria you can employ, but for reasons we will explore, they provide the best platform for competitive measurement and organizational prioritization.

In the past, I was fairly strident about the need for strict data-driven definition and classification. As it has played out over the years, however, I have modified my recommendation due to a number of factors, not the least of which is the sizeable hurdle that some organizations face in identifying the appropriate criteria for SL definition. For a large number of organizations, the strict data classifications are augmented by other criteria, such as net revenue as they measure it, overall volume, and, of course, net operating income.

Include OP Activity

Another complicating factor is the dramatic shift to OP procedures and visits. For most hospitals and health systems, the percentage of nonacute (also called ambulatory or OP) activity in both overall volume and net revenue has shifted from around 25% to 35% in the late nineties to 40% in the early 2000s to upward of 50% as of 2013. For some organizations, the relative proportion of OP activity is even higher.

Clearly, hospitals or health systems that define their SLs solely by DRGs/MS-DRGs (which are IP-based) see an incomplete picture of overall performance, since they are measuring only a declining segment of SL activity.

Refer to Figure 5.1 for an illustration of the growth of IP revenues over a 20 year period.

Figure 5.1| Growth of outpatient activity over time

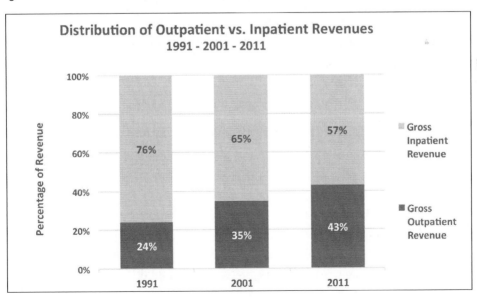

You will find that vendors (whether consultants, data management firms, or software platforms) have become much more astute and accurate in their ability to measure OP volume, activity, and financial performance, although it is still not as precise as it could and should be. Even hospitals and health systems without robust cost accounting platforms or decision support systems can outsource their data gathering and configuration to such firms, which can approximate fairly accurately the financial performance of the core SLs. And a couple of information management firms have recently partnered with claims data management enterprises to provide actual (not estimated) OP data.

2. Determine How to Assess Success (What Matters Should Get Measured)

Once you've established the criteria for determining how SLs will be defined, the next step is to determine which metrics matter most for your organization's key stakeholders. This is unlikely to be a difficult exercise, but it should prove illuminating to quantify the measures for each SL.

By metrics, I'm referring to measurable statistics or quantifiable components that determine the success or failure of the organization. These are the fundamentals that are reported to the board of directors, the community leaders, senior management, or whatever group is responsible for evaluating the ongoing success of your hospital or health system.

Financial metrics

Obviously, your organization's important financial indicator(s) should be included in this group. These include net income, operating margin, net patient revenue, and so forth.

As elementary as this may sound, I continue to be surprised and somewhat baffled that many provider organizations have not clarified, even among the senior leaders, which financial metrics matter most. Until the decision regarding financial metrics is rock solid and clearly communicated throughout the organization, it will be difficult to gauge the ultimate performance and success at the SL level. The key to effectiveness in this area is to have something that can be measured for each SL. In some cases (i.e., investor-owned facilities), the economic metric might be earnings before interest, taxes, depreciation, and amortization (EBITDA). Since this is the gauge that matters most to most for-profit hospitals, it makes absolute sense to take that level of financial performance down to the SL level.

Volume measures

You will also need one or more volume measures to effectively and competitively measure SL performance, such as total discharges for an IP consideration, or number of tests or surgeries for the OP component of the SL. You might also include a relative volume gauge, such as market share or market growth, for the particular SL or lines that are deemed as core to the organization.

One critical metric that is too often overlooked or discounted altogether is the relative performance on a volume basis against competitors. The ability to measure relative SL position (volume trends, preference, market share, etc.) against identified competitors is one of the main reasons for selecting definition criteria that are quantifiable and transferable across facilities within the market and even throughout the nation. Without data-driven categorization and definition of SLs, how can an organization and its leaders know if they are making any progress toward achieving their stated goals and objectives relative to their competitors?

Quality indicators

Other metrics to include are those providing quality indicators, such as complications or mortality indices. As with market share measures, these can be measured relative to area competitors or peer group hospitals within the industry (yet another reason for using quantifiable criteria in defining the SLs).

Such gauges of quality are becoming increasingly relevant as regional employer coalitions or national associations, such as The Leapfrog Group, become more involved in the operational component of the industry. Involvement and scrutiny by outside entities and key stakeholders will only intensify in the near future; be prepared to meet the demands of such groups with accurate and meaningful performance measures.

Market-facing metrics

With the rise of consumer engagement and the shift to a digital era, the metrics your organization chooses need to become more market facing. Measurements that were once not even on the radar screen will soon be critical for assessing the impact of potential success for an SL.

For example, one valuable market-facing metric might be visits to the organization's website, specific to a particular service, and click through on particular programs or services for that SL. This data will serve as a leading indicator for future business by consumers/patients, and it will also help you gauge the success of particular marketing campaigns or outreach efforts dedicated to a particular strategy for that SL. Just ask marketing professionals and SL leaders in other industries how important digital activity and ongoing measurement are to them, and you'll get a glimpse of where our industry and core metrics are heading and where our focus will need to be.

In summary, the list of success measures for SLs would include:

- IP volume for the SL (as measured by DRG classification or another comparable measure).

- OP visits, tests, procedures, or other relevant measures that are part of that SL offering.

- An overall volume metric that combines IP and OP. For example, some systems have developed an aggregate measure that equates OP volume to IP volume. One large faith-based system in the upper Midwest called this adjusted equivalent patient discharges (AEPD).

- Net revenue for the entire line—and also broken out by IP and OP.

- Contribution margin (net revenue minus direct costs).

- Net operating income (NOI). This is the term nonprofit organizations use, while the for-profit systems use EBDITA.

- Market metrics. Submeasures for success include customer relationship management (CRM) campaigns, visits to the Web page, click-throughs on the Web page, etc. These metrics are typically focused on marketing and outreach tactics, but they can be a useful part of the periodic reporting to key stakeholder groups. These will become not only an important leading indication of current and future volume, but a metric of keen interest to savvy senior leaders.

3. Narrow Down the Number of Lines to a Manageable Few

Your next step is to narrow the SLs down to a manageable number or to the critical few. The core SLs can be identified and singled out using the metrics identified in the previous step. You can work through this process using a series of analytical matrices and a variety of data-dependent graphs and tools, a few of which will be described in greater detail in Chapter 8.

The narrowing of SLs is a crucial step for a few reasons. First, it makes the implementation of SLM much easier to accomplish (or improve). Too many organizations begin the SL process and organization with too many SLs.

They're not all core

I once worked with a hospital that had identified 23 SLs. When I asked them which of this vast number were priorities, the CEO said, "All of them."

There's nothing inherently wrong with eventually having more than three or four SLs that represent the organization's main efforts (although 23 was too many, and always will be); the critical activity here is to focus on only the truly significant strategic business units (SLs) that can and will differentiate the organization competitively and improve its overall market position.

I have found that organizations that are unable to definitively identify those three or four core SLs lack planning clarity and focus or suffer a general uncertainty as to where the organization is really focusing its resources, or both. Such organizations also tend to vacillate, shifting SL priorities and reacting more to extraneous factors (e.g., prominent physician pet projects, board member influence, competitor moves, etc.) rather than responding to clearly defined market need and data-driven long-term planning objectives.

The second reason for focusing on no more than four SLs is management's attention and resource commitment. For example, if an organization identifies 10 lines that are going to demand management time and attention, in reality and execution, the entire effort will be diffused. Those 10 lines are just too many plates to keep spinning, so to speak.

When you are first implementing your SL strategies, it is far better to identify just two, three, or (at the most) four SLs that can realistically be monitored, managed, and differentiated from a competitive standpoint. This prioritization needs to be undertaken at the highest level of the organization and thoroughly communicated and understood at the crucial midrange level, where the core accountability will likely reside.

Here's the deal: When you narrow the focus of the organization down to just a few strategic business units, upper management can invest time and expend resources to staff those SLs with dedicated people. This narrowing down and high-profile focus approach has proven far more effective than piling one more responsibility onto an already overworked middle manager or administrative-level executive.

The latter dynamic (of adding additional responsibility to an already-stretched middle manager) is much more likely to occur if the organization has identified more than four SLs, because virtually every hospital and health system in the nation is now under a strict mandate to restrict the hiring of new or additional personnel to a minimum. Hiring an outside manager for each SL, or even elevating an existing manager with dedicated time and resources to that SL responsibility, will not be met with much enthusiasm if the organization has identified too many SLs.

The notion of organizing a matrix team (the optimal configuration for an SL structure, discussed in detail in Chapter 9) for each SL has produced very favorable results for many hospitals. Yet the identification and deployment of effective matrix teams is far less likely to occur when the hospital or health system has five or more identified strategic business units (SBU) at the outset of its SL implementation. Again, it just stretches already-busy people to the max.

Apply the Pareto Principle

Many companies outside healthcare have become more successful with a product line or SL approach by following the Pareto Principle, or the 80/20 rule. This rule of thumb asserts that roughly 80% of an organization's successful performance (however that is measured) is derived from approximately 20% of its products or services. The healthcare industry will be well served to understand and more artfully apply this time-tested principle of management.

The best way to identify the core SLs is by applying a Pareto approach to an objective measurement of your current SLs. Once you establish the metrics that matter, you can then use them to prioritize the SLs. For example, a simple two-axis grid can graphically display the three or four SLs that provide the bulk of the organization's net revenues, contribution margin, and net operating income.

Alternatively, the organization may to focus on other metrics, such as market perception by the consumer, strong medical staff, or high quality scores in particular SLs. The metrics that matter most for your key stakeholders will inform the data, and the application of the Pareto Principle will identify your strongest SLs.

Typical top lines

For most mid- to large-size hospitals, the three or four line SLs that usually account for between 60% to 75% of the enterprise's net revenue are among this list: general medicine, general surgery, orthopedics, cardiovascular (CV), oncology, women's services, and, sometimes, neurosciences. In contrast, the five leading lines (for the majority of mid- to large-size hospitals) that account for between 50% and 70% of the net operating income are usually general surgery, orthopedics, CV, oncology (particularly if radiation therapy is significant), and neurosciences (if offered).

These comparative statistics don't necessarily hold true for all organizations, but they do for well over half of mid- to large-size hospitals.

Figure 5.2 | The Pareto principle applied to SLM

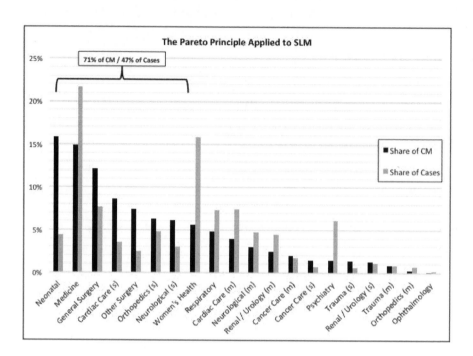

4. Establish the Optimal Managerial Team

Once the number of SLs has been narrowed to three or four core lines that are pivotal to your organization's success, the next step is to establish the managerial team. Having narrowed your focus to a small number of crucial lines, it will be much easier to identify the right individuals and the proper organizational construct for those high-priority SLs.

There are many variables to consider in this process, but one of the first that organizations should grapple with is the internal versus external candidate decision. Based on my observations, the success of the model is more a function of attitude and personality than it is of "insiders" versus "outsiders." For example, some internal candidates with entrepreneurial flair have made excellent SL managers. You'll also need to consider the ever-important issue of organizational dynamics and stakeholder considerations.

Still, there are pros and cons to internal versus external candidates. For an SL that relies heavily on particular physician specialties, an established clinical manager—one who enjoys a stellar reputation and outstanding rapport with the doctors—may be the logical candidate. On the other hand, intense or changing local market dynamics may call for someone who brings fresh perspective and creative approaches to an SL that has been stagnant and needs rejuvenation.

As noted earlier, the migration to a consumer-driven healthcare model will demand a particularly market-savvy individual in the role of SL overseer and choreographer. The organization will want someone who understands the role of digital media in market-facing communication and data analytics. This is relatively new territory for our industry, so few managers and directors (at least at the SL level) have experience in this area. That noted, if you find a great SL candidate or even existing manager without digital media experience, the right individual can learn.

The other critical organizational issue is the support group that backs up the dedicated manager or director of the SL. This can be a task force (an ad hoc group), a matrix team (more permanent in nature), or a hybrid of the two. Whatever the design, each SL should include individuals representing a wide array of related functional areas that provide input and insight into the operational component of the SL.

5. Evaluate Market Position by SL

Once the organizational design is determined and the individuals responsible for managing and building the lines are in place, the organization will need to perform a competitive assessment.

You may have difficulty executing on this particular phase of implementation, due to cost accounting constraints within the system, or data limitations within the region, but the competitive assessment is critical to a successful SL approach. During this phase of the process, you'll assess your newly identified core SLs against those of the most relevant competitive organization(s) within your market to serve as important market gauges or benchmarks. These comparative benchmarks (i.e., competitive organizations) may be peer groups (similar size and services throughout the state or nation) or local/regional competition. Most of the time, local and regional competitors are more relevant, but for some hospitals and health systems that compete on a broader geographic basis, competitors within the state or even in other parts of the country may provide a valid benchmark.

The metrics used to make the competitive market assessment should certainly include those categories identified in step two above—"measure what matters"— but it also could involve additional measures that might be relevant to that particular SL and the specific market dynamic.

For example, the competitive assessment would likely include several qualitative measures, such as public surveys that measure awareness and quality perception, as well as many measures that include a more broad-range assessment by several of the key stakeholder groups—especially physicians. Several of these measures (and how to derive them) are discussed later in the book, which provides more information on this facet of SL execution.

The competitive assessment is important for a number of obvious reasons, not the least of which is capital allocation. In these times of constrained capacity and restricted capital, many hospitals must make difficult decisions when it comes to the allocation of capital. One of the most daunting is which expansion or development opportunities are best suited for the long-range success of the organization. These significant capital spending decisions should never be made without a thorough understanding of how individual services are positioned— perceptually and strategically—against competitors, both existing and potential. For example, I have seen hospitals and health systems undertake major capital expansion for particular SLs (renovated wing, new center of excellence, etc.) without realistically factoring in the strength of and relative position of existing competition. The old days of "build it and they will come" are long since over, and just offering the service or ramping it up most certainly does not guarantee its ultimate success.

That said, there is definite value in preemptive or even sometimes strong, calculated defensive moves, if they are well-positioned and market-changing. This is the area where the discussion of niche players, specialty hospitals, and physician ventures comes into play the most. One of the best arguments for developing or strengthening the SL structure is to counter or preempt these new competitors, which are threatening to erode the economic core of many larger hospitals and health systems in the country.

6. Develop Business Plans for Each SL that Syncs with the Strategic Plan

Once the competitive assessment is completed, develop a business plan for each SL. Some organizations include the competitive assessment as the introductory element of the SL business plan—in the environmental analysis section. That decision is entirely up to management, and much depends on how the individual business plans and the more broad-based strategic plan have been developed within the organization in the past.

A caution related to business planning

Resist the temptation to spend so much time on the environmental assessment or market analysis that the market backdrop becomes the main focus of the planning effort.

Here's why: Having sat through and presented innumerable strategic/business plan presentations, I can tell you that by the time audiences have heard and tried to absorb the endless array of data and statistics in the environmental analysis, they are so worn out that they often want to speed right through the objectives and strategies, which results in suboptimal business planning.

A better approach: Separate the environmental assessment segment of the plan discussion and presentation from the strategy and goal-setting segment(s) of the planning process. I have seen this done effectively by organizations and consultants who recognize the value in providing *just enough* framework for a leadership team or board to then develop the requisite and appropriate road map to advance the strategic direction of their enterprise.

The **objectives segment** of any business or strategic plan should demand the most time and focus, for that is what will drive the organization's resource allocation and ultimately determine its successful trajectory. Yet, the objectives and strategies often are derived in haste or frustration rather than deliberated at length and revisited for reasonableness. The plan that often emerges from rushing through definition of the objectives is more operational or tactical than truly strategic in nature.

Strategies are those elegant statements of action that should be well planned and thoughtfully, deliberately executed. Each major strategy should come under concerted scrutiny. Each strategy should pass the litmus test in its ability to help achieve the objective or goal with which it is associated and, accordingly, improve the operating position of the overall organization. Metaphorically speaking, if an inordinate amount of time is spent on the frame of a painting (in this case, the environmental analysis), few individuals will have the patience—or the endurance—to appreciate the brushstrokes on the canvas.

Eventually, the business plan must get down to the minute details, but this level of **granularity** is best presented in an appendix or otherwise kept in the background. Although important, such managerial and tactical "minutiae" can be colossally distracting. The granular details should be left to the individuals responsible for successful implementation of the specifics and never reviewed with key decision-makers or stakeholder groups, such as the board, medical staff members, or senior management. If the board or even executive management is that deeply into the "weeds," then the organization is headed for trouble.

Nonetheless, it is good to have that level of granularity in writing and available for reference, and for accountability's sake.

7. Compete Strategically at the Micromarket Level

One difference between SLM in the new consumer-driven climate compared to earlier periods is a reduced emphasis on certain facets of execution. The first wave of service/product line management became so focused on external execution elements—promotion and marketing—that they overshadowed the organizational aspect.

Emphasizing a focus on the micromarket (key stakeholder or customer) by no means diminishes the significance of an effective and well-targeted marketing and promotional strategy. Rather, the broader point is to put the organizational building blocks of definition, design, execution, and so forth into clear focus. In other words, if all those aspects are done and done well, then the promotional/communication phase will have a higher probability of achieving the overall objective, which positions the organization in a more competitive way.

The nature of competition has changed in the past few years. As explored throughout the book, healthcare organizations (particularly providers) face much savvier competitors, with greater understanding of the customer and a heightened ability to communicate and speak his or her language. This ramped-up competition requires not only increased sophistication in design of the delivery model and delivery of the message but, importantly, a refined understanding of the nature of the targeted stakeholder segment. In essence, you will need a much greater focus on listening and learning—via market research.

Thorough market research is not an area where very many healthcare organizations have achieved (or even attempted to achieve) much success. Yet to prevail over the new wave of competitors, tried and true methodology used in effective market research must be employed, and the information then deployed in the design and implementation of the organization's strategy.

8. Update the Model Periodically to Reflect Market Changes

Once the organization has applied the SL model and demonstrated that it is viable and invaluable, the key is to keep the SL approach dynamic and the design current.

We already have seen a high degree of modification in the application of SLs within this field, as the market has shifted to adopt new configurations and adjustments. As we enter a landscape of dramatically empowered and engaged consumers, it is critical to keep the SL model in sync with the changing environment. This is the capstone rule for two reasons.

First, it conveys to the entire organization that there is fluidity in the organizational approach to the market.

Second, it shows that this (i.e., SLM) is an initiative that is integral to the ongoing operation of the hospital or health system and that as the market changes, competitors emerge, and opportunities present, the managerial model for dealing with those challenges and opportunities will align with the changing landscape.

Conclusion

The key to the success of the steps outlined above is to ensure that, coupled with their adoption, there is a commitment to adaptability and agility as appropriate to the individual market.

This essential flexibility hinges on one of the first steps—designing the model with just a few SLs. By proving out the concept with just two to four SLs, the organization is actually in a much better position to align the model with the market and to successfully apply the structure within the confines of organizational dynamics, appropriately aligning enterprise strengths with market demands. In other words, it's easier to steer a small vessel than the organizational equivalent of a supertanker.

Ironically, the organization attempting to implement the model in a nonprioritized, or broader sense (e.g., over five or more SLs) is more likely to abandon the SL model before it can be fully vetted and validated. History tells us that given the still-nascent nature of an SL structure in many healthcare organizations, incremental implementation and execution provide a much more likely road to higher performance.

These are the fundamental steps in understanding and implementing an SL model. If adopted, incorporated, and followed, they can facilitate a successful adaptation of the managerial model that has worked for countless firms in multiple industries. I'll describe most of these steps in greater detail in subsequent chapters.

6

Defining
Service Lines
in the New World Order

Why Definitions Are so Crucial

Hospitals and health systems often get bogged down on one of the first steps
in successful service line (SL) structure and strategy: defining what constitutes
an SL. As important as this step is, it can derail the initial momentum when
managers prolong the struggle to place parameters on the nature of SLs within the
organization.

To implement service line management (SLM) successfully, you will need to
prioritize your SLs. However, prioritization can only occur when SLs are defined
in a way that makes it possible to compare data, both within the organization and
throughout the market.

Functional Parameters Require Good Data

If a hospital defines SLs based on criteria that are too specific, assessment will
be difficult. For that reason, even though more hospitals are creating subset SLs,

such as bariatric surgery (a subset of general surgery) or radiation therapy (a subset of the oncology SL) it will be well worth the effort to establish ground rules for clear definition. It should begin at a higher or broader level (i.e., cardiovascular or orthopedics SL as the categories), prior to subdividing or defining them too narrowly.

The problem with narrow and project-oriented structural definitions is simple: These approaches usually lack comparative data sources to measure market success. Without data that can be measured within the organization, managers cannot determine the relative value of a particular segment, and therefore they cannot perform the critical task of prioritization.

Priorities must be established to ensure that limited capital is being allocated to SLs where it will have the greatest return. Organizational resources also need to be parceled out based on the overriding organizational strategy, which will be determined in large part by the relative strength of each area—financial and operational.

Hybrid or Second-Stage SLs

Some hospitals and health systems use a looser definition of SLs, and that can work depending on the organization, the local market dynamics, and a host of other factors. Prior to pursuing these nontraditional categorizations, or offshoots of the traditional SL definition, however, it's best to establish your standard SLM format and model. If this step isn't accomplished, namely establishing the traditional framework with standard definitions and so forth, it will be very difficult to effectively monitor progress against competitive benchmarks for the overall SL model. Accordingly, I recommend that the organization develop the model with traditional definitions of SLs (oncology, cardiovascular services, etc.) before using a hybrid or nontraditional SL definition (i.e., wellness, men's health, etc.).

After creating the larger SL framework, some organizations pursue alternative approaches, some of which might include:

- A service that actually is a subset of an SL (as described above), such as bariatric surgery. The SL is general surgery, and the bariatric subsegment eventually can be isolated and monitored on its own. This particular service sub-segment is a popular SL category, especially for marketers, as it is very consumer facing, is easily tracked for return on investment (ROI), and typically realizes a high correlation between promotional expenses and increased volume.

- A department or function that does not produce revenue reimbursed by commercial or government payers but is rather more of a retail operation. An example of this would be a spa. Another popular "SL" is a fitness center. These services usually rely more heavily on cash or out-of-pocket reimbursement, so the standard framework and definitions don't apply that neatly to such SLs, but they certainly can be measured based on other criteria, and many hospitals choose to do so. And a number of the steps discussed previously in establishing effective SLs apply here, including the development of a business plan, the establishment of a matrix team, and the use of market research to gauge consumer interests and preferences.

- An umbrella category that touches a number of SL categories, but is so broad that it is difficult to actually measure, such as "medical services." This SL is not to be confused with "general medicine," (which has standard definitional criteria, such as DRGs, ICD, etc.). Rather, as I have sometimes seen it defined, "medical services" is even broader than the general medicine SL, and involves several medicine-related SLs, such as medical cardiology, medical oncology, and so forth. The difficulty with this type of broad classification lies in the comparative measures against competitors, as well as a general mish-mash of the other traditional SL definitions and categorizations. For that reason, I usually recommend against broad, umbrella classifications or designations.

- Services that may be interesting and in vogue but difficult to track and measure. An example of this is complementary and alternative medicine (CAM), or what is also referred to as integrative medicine.

A caution about defining CAM as an SL

Although things have changed in recent years, I learned from my experience at St. David's HealthCare (a partnership with HCA) about integrative medicine. For a brief time, I served as the chair of the CAM task force for HCA and conducted a fair amount of research into the area. What I learned then still holds true to large extent—for most systems and in most areas, CAM/integrative medicine lacks substantive benchmark data for comparison, as well as an effective means to assess reimbursement criteria. Integrative medicine may be worth pursuing as a viable service category for some hospitals or health systems, but its inability to fit succinctly into the typical definitions and framework of the other SLs will prove problematic. That said, many of the core elements of SL planning (business plans, market research, multifunction matrix teams, etc.) can readily apply to an effective and successful integrative medicine offering. CAM might be considered in a unique strategic business segment, but I caution against infusing it into the mix during the early stages of SL development, as it will likely confuse the general design and implementation of the overall SL application.

Some health executives might dismiss my recommendation for this approach, as they have established SLs that fall into these categories. I do recognize that a number of organizations have established similar strategic business segments as SLs, but it is generally more effective to establish SLs with a framework that allows for comparative evaluation and data-driven assessment, and later incorporate the less traditional lines of business within the SL construct.

I have observed that sometimes the management team first determines what SLs they want to offer based on criteria outside of the standard framework I described earlier (uniform and data-driven definitions and so forth) and uses that criteria to designate service segments or department function as SLs. This approach doesn't provide adequate consideration for the overall framework of the SL model and its applicability in the broader sense. It is extremely important for senior executives to view SLM as the framework to assess the organization's viability and performance in the context of the competitive market.

If the leadership of the organization adopts an SL model that pivots its design off a nontraditional, difficult-to-measure SL (e.g., wellness services), they lose the more important ability to assess competitive performance in their core SLs, such as cardiovascular, general surgery, orthopedics, oncology, and neurosciences. Those SLs likely account for 75% of hospital (or health system) net revenue and net operating income and accordingly should form the basis of the SL model design. Otherwise, it's a proverbial case of the tail wagging the dog.

The fundamental issue with using a nontraditional SL to form the basis of the overall model is that the management team runs the risk of implementing a business/strategic plan without analyzing the mission-critical business segments of the enterprise within the context of the emerging competitive environment. In essence, they are allowing the nominal to override the dominant. I have seen this happen too often, largely because it is easier to discuss and review services that have a simpler definition and organizational reporting structure (e.g., retail services) than deal with SLs that are difficult to define and measure and even more difficult to administer and grow (e.g., oncology). But complexity and difficulty should not deter executive leaders from tackling the challenge of defining, managing, and monitoring the SLs that will determine the long-term viability of the organization. That is why you start with the Pareto group and then branch out from there. Having objectively determined the areas of greatest value, the organization will appropriately allocate resources and management time to the most crucial areas.

Optimally, your crucial "value" and priority determination may be based on criteria ranging from financial to mission fulfillment, and I recommend that you employ relative measures of market strength and long-term success, as well as objective data that can be measured and reviewed over time.

As we move toward a more consumer-driven model, with less room for error and more pressure on the bottom line, choosing strategic business units or SLs that are only moderate performers, or that don't necessarily offer the organization a breakout opportunity for success, will not only diminish the organization's strategic position in the market, it may result in a serious competitive disadvantage.

That said, if a hybrid or second-stage SL strategy is working for your organization, and your management team has done an effective job of prioritizing the SLs that matter most, then whom am I to suggest fixing what isn't broken? Don't disrupt the market karma.

The Role of Data in the Process

A good SL approach should serve two vital purposes: streamlining your strategy and focusing your resources. If it does not achieve those fundamental objectives, then the truth is, the existing structure is suboptimal.

The only way these two core objectives can be realized is through the use of consistent, accurate, comparative data. As noted earlier, one of the first steps in executing a successful SL model is determining the criteria for identifying the SLs. At that point, you will apply the criteria you've chosen to establish relative measures.

To that end I strongly recommend using the following data-related criteria for establishing benchmark measures to define your SLs.

DRG or MS-DRG data

Historically, the most common such measure has been the diagnosis-related group (DRG), or hospital inpatient payment methodology, data configuration for the definition of inpatient lines. One of the key reasons for using a DRG-based architecture (at least at the outset) is the availability and comparability of data within the market (with hospital competitors) and across the SLs within the organization.

Interestingly, this was not always the case. When SLs were first being developed, the data configurations were not robust, and data sources were limited. However, in recent years, several data-repository healthcare firms have emerged, either through the merger of competing or comparable firms or through organic growth. These firms now offer a wider complement of services with deeper concentration and broader geographic reach in their comparative data banks.

Changes in DRG definition/configuration since the last edition

In the fall of 2009, the classification index was changed by the Centers for Medicare and Medicaid Services (CMS) to Medicare severity-adjusted diagnosis related groups (MS-DRGs), and the number of disease categories, which is modified fairly frequently, increased to the 800 range, in contrast to the original 400+ when DRGs were first introduced in 1983.

It is important to recognize that, despite the fact that most people in the industry still use the term DRG rather than MS-DRG, this new classification index has significantly impacted the definitions of SLs due to the revised disease categories and SL groupings. Most of the data firms that provide SL definitions use MS-DRGs, but some of the health systems in the country (particularly the for-profit systems) use their own definitions and groupings for SLs, rendering comparisons across competitors difficult to assess. However, most SL data experts can provide close approximations, as can the data-based firms that provide the core definitions for the systems which are their clients.

All that said, if the SL definitions haven't been revisited and revised for a few years (especially since the introduction of MS-DRGs), hospitals and health systems already practicing SL management should take this opportunity to review and recalibrate, as the expanded classifications may well require a reconstitution of SLs. Along with the practical implications of the DRG reconfiguration, there are the strategic ramifications for the new structure (such as the reduced reimbursement for the procedural categories and the increased payments for medical areas). Whatever your situation, this significant change in disease category classification should provide a window of opportunity for all health systems to either evaluate or reevaluate the SL construct within their organization.

Regardless of the impact of this relatively recent configuration, one significant challenge for some SLs is the inherent complexity of a particular SL category. For example, oncology is among the most challenging SLs to define. This is due to many factors, not the least of which is the cross-categorization of particular procedures and diagnoses—that is, a number of the diagnoses and procedures that realistically could fall into any number of designated SLs.

So what sources exist for data today? There are a few options available:

- Perhaps the easiest and most workable solution is to use definitions provided by **national data firms** (i.e., Health Care Advisory Board, Sg2, Truven, and others) and apply the same classification of DRGs/MS-DRGs as they do.

- Another option is to do what several hospitals have done with reasonable success, which is to apply **majority-rule criteria**, meaning the appropriate SL for each DRG is determined by the percentage of organization-specific cases based on the primary diagnosis. For example, if a particular DRG has 51% of the diagnoses that are cancer-related, then all of the admissions for that DRG accrue to the oncology SL. There are a number of organizations that use this model, as imperfect as it may seem. And while this approach may not seem sufficiently accurate or even representative, I have recommended this approach a few times, as such a definitive decision is needed to move the organization beyond analysis paralysis which would render it unable to define the SL parameters at all.

- Another method many healthcare organizations employ is to keep different sets of books for SL measurement. For example, one savvy SL system used standard definitions from one of the national database firms (in this case The Advisory Board) to array its SL performance against its local competitor. At the same time, they used different definitions/classifications for two specific SLs (in this case, trauma and oncology) because they felt the national definitions didn't adequately capture the full scope of the performance of those two services lines for internal comparisons and resource allocation. This may sound rather complex, but it actually worked well for this system, as they had an "external" definition (to compare performance in the market) and an "internal" definition to compare intra-company.

A caution about assigning DRGs/MS-DRGs to complex SLs

The truth is that there aren't many SLs with diagnoses (or DRGs) that fall into a gray area. Most diagnoses clearly align with one particular SL, which makes assigning them to the correct SL a relatively uncomplicated task. However, determining the appropriate bucket in which to place more challenging DRGs can prove frustrating, even to the point of an impasse for some organizations.

The important thing is to get beyond hand-wringing and head-scratching relative to the problematic DRGs and move on to the stage of organizationwide analysis. And since there are only one or two SLs for which these challenging DRGs come into play (primarily oncology), you needn't allow them to become a show-stopper. The fact is that detailed definition and category assignments can always be modified later in the process, as data collection improves and the actual execution of strategy takes shape. In other words, don't let perfect become the enemy of good.

Once the definitions have been solidified and you have clarified which DRGs fall within the identified SLs, it's time to gather the data on each line. Many organizations have the capacity to conduct this analysis with their existing resources. If not, they can tap into the resources of outside data management firms with which they are already contracted. Increasingly, hospitals and health systems are outsourcing data gathering and data arraying functionality to firms that have deep data repositories and sophisticated data analytical capability. In certain states, there are also database resources that compile, array, and distribute the data to client members.

In some instances, these entities are subsidiaries or departments of the state hospital association, so the data gathering and configuration tends to be statewide. In other instances, these organizations have a narrower geographic scope, such as a large metro area, where hospitals and health systems have banded together to make the data available and to share the cost to do so. The advantage of the more limited geographic entities often comes down to timing of data release and availability.

Internal vs. external data resources

Interestingly, I have found that many senior leaders are unaware of the data resources to which they already have access and the kinds of reports that can be generated from internal data sources.

A first step in determining how to assemble and array internal data is to ask your Information Services (IS), financial, and perhaps planning staff what is available through existing resources, such as the cost accounting system, purchased data management, or even systemwide reports. Some systems maintain a proprietary database that closely parallels a chosen data repository's SL classification.

Next, you may want to engage a data firm. Assess who your competition uses, as well as how your own internal resources (i.e., the decision support system) align with the prospective data firm's definitions and process for data gathering. Several leading data firms have merged in recent years, resulting in more uniform and universal definitions. Even among larger firms, however, you will still find differences in how they define SLs and what measurement criteria they use, so pay attention to those differences as you make your selection.

You'll find great advantages in using this type of resource, including the ability to gauge the performance of the SLs against local, regional, and national competition. But some of the hospitals and health systems that might consider their organizations to be in the SL mode have not yet overcome the problem of having ineffective or insufficient measurement capabilities. I continue to be surprised that a fair number of health systems, including some of the largest in the country, still have inadequate or virtually nonexistent cost accounting structures and decision support systems. I find it mind-boggling to think that a multibillion dollar enterprise would not be able to accurately monitor and manage its financial performance at the strategic business unit level. In my mind, it is nothing short of essential to have an effective decision support system and cost accounting structure that enables you to conduct a thorough, accurate analysis of their internal portfolio by SLs.

The acute need for accurate cost accounting at the SL level will only intensify as we face the emerging environment of empowered and engaged consumers, who will want to know the costs of their services and the value they're deriving for those expenditures.

Drill Down on the Data

If for no other reason than to effectively assess the level of prioritized reimbursement, it is worthwhile to do a sophisticated SL review. Since DRGs/MS-DRGs are the operative classification for getting reimbursed from the government for inpatient procedures (through Medicare and Medicaid), a data-defined SL model enables the SL manager and the team responsible for each SL to analyze the financial appropriateness of each individual DRG, as well as the line in its entirety.

Unfortunately, due to the general nature of SL structure, many hospitals and health systems never get to that level of granularity. However, if the SL team can be organized and function properly, then the value of having a full complement of departments and organizational expertise can be brought to bear in assessing the detailed reimbursement picture. I was first made aware of this reality when I entered the realm of healthcare (from the packaged goods industry) at Sacred Heart Hospital in Eugene, Oregon. One of the first things we did in our SL teams was to conduct a DRG by DRG financial assessment. This was quite illuminating for all of us, but particularly for the physicians involved in our SL matrix team. That was a number of years ago, and that level of granular analysis has become even more critical today, as government reimbursement continues to be ratcheted down, and the number of treatments, procedures, tests, and care protocols that generate a positive net margin gets smaller and smaller.

Once a line has been defined, the SL team can evaluate each DRG classification on a modified contribution basis to determine whether the reimbursement from the government is sufficient to cover the costs and meet the financial goals of the hospital. When that analysis is underway, the SL director (along with the entire team) can begin to develop and implement strategies on a collective or even individual DRG basis (or, for outpatient, on an Ambulatory Payment Classification basis) that factors in the reimbursement consideration.

Obviously, this kind of granular drill-down by procedural code or category is much more readily accomplished when the SLs are defined by data classifications. That is just one of several good reasons for defining the lines based on data divisions.

Picturing the lines

The process of arraying the lines can be quite instructive. Relevant data for the identified SLs should be first assembled, then verified, then arrayed. There are several ways to array the data, but the best methods are those that involve easily understandable and compelling graphics.

For example, a portfolio grid can display a vast amount of data along two (or perhaps three) evaluative criteria. Figure 6.1 presents data on 16 SLs using three variables: market share, projected SL growth rate, and CM per case.

In this figure, the y axis is a depiction of the market share for that particular SL. The size of the bubble depicts the margin per case (or discharge in this instance, since this graph is for inpatient volume). This metric is a good financial gauge that is relevant to every hospital and health system, and such a graphic depiction allows key stakeholder (SL matrix team, executive management, board of directors, etc.) a snapshot visual of the relative bottom-line position of each of the organization's major SLs. The x axis measures market growth potential for each of the SLs on the graph for the next five years. A growth measure is highly relevant and useful as it provides a view of future state opportunity and comes into play in assessing resource allocation and capital expenditures. In this case, the data are drawn from a national source, but this measurement can also be based on either historical data or projections. Either way, the growth coefficient is critical, because whereas the other two measures provide a current state view, this element gives a sense of the SL's potential.

Figure 6.1| Service line portfolio grid

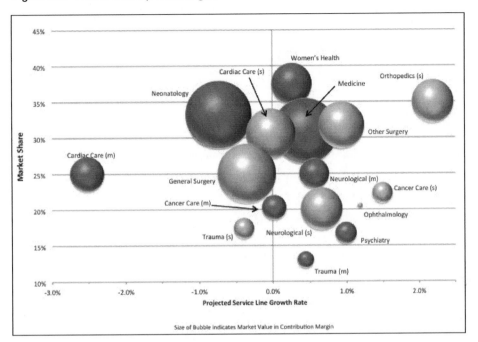

Size of Bubble indicates Market Value in Contribution Margin

A line may have stellar financial performance but exist in a climate of stagnant growth potential. For example, in this grid, the neonatal line has a very high contribution margin per case but is actually in a negative growth position in this market. In a case like this, you might argue for a strategy of protecting current volumes, but this organization may not have sufficient rationale for committing sizable resources or capital to the neonatal SL, since the growth potential is limited. Given the nature of the neonatal SL and its limited competitive threat (in some markets at least), the low-growth (or declining growth in this cast) may prompt a strategy of expanding the market to a regional or even state-wide span.

Other SLs may indicate the potential for significant growth but not offer the promise of attractive margins. In this graphic, we can see that dynamic with ophthalmology and psychiatry, both of which have fairly good growth potential, but on a relative scale have lower than average contribution margins per case. Data such as that shown in our example may foreshadow the SL's diminishment, future consolidation, or even closure. More than a few hospitals and health systems have used similar graphs to assess the long-term viability of SLs.

In fact, when I consulted with systems and individual hospitals, it was often a revealing snapshot such as this that prompted senior management to review its overall portfolio of offerings and, in some case, determine that one or two SLs should no longer be in the mix. In more than one instance, for example, obstetrics was eliminated from the portfolio following an analysis that began with a relative market positioning graph like this one. Alternatively, the lower-margin SLs may also highlight a need for operational improvements or efficiencies, or more accurate coding of procedures, or they may simply indicate that reimbursement is not keeping up with the overhead related to delivering the service.

In the case where reimbursement has not kept pace with the resources required to deliver the care, key players in the organization may have the data you need to lobby payers to reimburse more in line with the costs of the procedure and associated organizational resources.

Conclusion

Defining the SLs is an important first step in establishing an effective SL structure. If you execute poorly on the definition of your SLs, you run the risk of being unable to track performance. Loosely defined metrics and objectives don't provide the criteria for evaluating competitive performance and lack well-delineated accountability measures.

In short, ill-defined lines will simply not deliver the full value of the SL model to your enterprise and may well derail long-term implementation of your overarching strategy. To avoid that unfortunate outcome, the savvy SL director will pay particular attention to the manner in which the SLs are defined and will use a data-driven methodology offering objective quantification, internal prioritization, and ongoing competitive evaluation to do so.

7

Analytics, Anyone?

Defining the Metrics that Equate to Success

One of the key components often missing from the early stages of design
and development of service lines (SL) is the establishment of metrics for
gauging success. All too often, these metrics are identified further down the
implementation path. When treated as an afterthought, the measures are less
likely to be representative of and consistent with the organization's overarching
and long-range strategy. The result is a disjointed or even out-of-sync evaluation
of the SL performance relative to the rest of the organization. The SL model never
has the full opportunity to prove itself.

In one health system, for example, an SL manager was evaluated on his ability to
attract new patients to the SL with little consideration for that particular business
unit's operating margin. Consequently, he succeeded in increasing overall volume,
but in an SL of the hospital that had a low margin. The outcome was that the
operating margin for that particular SL deteriorated. At the same time, the

organizational resources, management focus, and financial capital allocated to the lower-margin SL drew limited resources away from higher margin lines, to the detriment of the overall financial position of the organization.

Applying a Mix of Both: Quantitative Measures

This anecdote illustrates the need for an organization to identify—early and definitively—metrics that align with the core objectives of managerial attention and will ensure the long-term viability of the organization. These measures should become the criteria for prioritizing the SLs, establishing objectives for each line, and ultimately evaluating the success of specific strategies outlined in each line's business plan.

Successful organizations know that it is well worth the effort to identify such measures at the outset. Then, when the time comes to develop SL business plans, the goals and strategies for each SL will more closely align with the organization's primary objectives.

For many organizations, most selected quantitative metrics will be financial in nature. These measures include net revenue, contribution margin, net operating income, or, in the case of for-profit entities, earnings before interest, taxes, depreciation, and amortization (EBITDA). Financial measures may also include days cash on hand, debt ratios, or other measures of liquidity.

Consideration also may be given to other balance sheet criteria that influence an organization's bond rating. In these times of diminishing reimbursement and reduced capital, bond rating metrics are increasingly important, as organizations are pressed to expand capacity to meet the increasing demands of an aging population. Consequently, access to the capital markets, which for many is via the bond route, will become increasingly critical. (Note: Some of the bond rating metrics, liquidity ratios, days cash on hand, and so forth can be difficult to translate down to the SL level, but extrapolations can be made where applicable.)

What is discussed in the C-Suite should be the SL metrics

In developing the list of metrics that matter most, senior leaders need to pose the question, *"What do we discuss the most at our executive leadership sessions and at our board meetings?"*

For most organizations, the answer to that question will be financial statements, economic measures, and, perhaps, competitive metrics such as market share or volume indicators. This is not always the case, but experience shows that much of the discussion in executive sessions and at board meetings centers on the subject of financial results and market measurements, even among faith-based organizations. This focus is not necessarily a negative thing; it is just a reality of the environment and the economic, regulatory, and competitive pressures that the provider sector faces.

Financial metrics

Within the category of financial measurements, however, the item that matters most will vary by market and type of organization.

- **EBITDA:** At investor-owned or for-profit hospitals, the statistic that gets the most attention is EBITDA, or *earnings before interest, taxes, depreciation, and amortization.* For many of the privately held companies, such as HCA, Tenet, Community Health Systems, and other for-profit chains, it probably is fair to say that this calculation receives as much attention as any other metric, which is understandable, as Wall Street also focuses on this measure of market viability. Spend any time in one of these organizations, and you quickly ascertain that this is the measure on which budgets are based and toward which business plans are oriented. Those who have worked in the for-profit sector know that EBITDA is thoroughly scrutinized and evaluated on a very frequent basis. The senior executives and mid-level managers in these organizations are intimately familiar with this measure, as it usually accounts for the lion's share of their incentive compensation.

- **Net operating income (NOI):** In the **nonprofit** world, on the other hand, the calculation that matters most is likely NOI, sometimes referred to as net margin. In the nonprofit world, the term "profit" is used sparingly, if at all.

More common is the term "margin" or NOI, depending on how the hospital or health system refers to its bottom line.

- **Contribution margin:** Some organizations like to gauge *contribution margin* (what's left over after direct or variable costs have been considered) to assess the organization's ability to contribute toward fixed or indirect costs.

- **Revenue:** A fair number of organizations will focus on *net revenue* as a critical measure. However, emphasis on revenue (usually net revenue—or what is collected—not gross revenue or "charges") is decreasing as executives recognize that not all volume is necessarily beneficial, depending on the nature of the payer mix. For example, a hospital may have a high percentage of self-pay and Medicaid patients, offset by a less-than-optimal percentage of commercially insured, such that it can barely stay afloat financially. In this increasingly common scenario (especially in urban hospitals) the margin considerations within the individual SLs play an even greater role in sustaining the viability of the organization. A decreasing number of organizations give serious consideration to the artificial top line of *gross revenue,* as it has little material value or relevance, except perhaps as a shadowboxing exercise to show what the organization "should have received" for the provision of its services. But few stakeholder groups or interested parties (including the media) care to hear that story anymore.

The financial metrics identified above have very likely been determined as essential for the organization in total. Consequently, these critical measures— which are the subject of extensive review and discussion at executive sessions and board meetings—should become the basis for evaluating performance at the SL level as well.

Competitive metrics

In the world of consumer-driven healthcare, some very important metrics have emerged that weren't even on the radar just a few years ago:

- **Website metrics:** As the industry moves into the digital realm, much like other consumer-driven organizations, the metric of *website visits* will become increasingly more prominent, along with **click-through rate**, which speaks to how many individuals dove deeper into the website content and then did something with the content.

- **Marketing metrics:** Along those lines, marketing metrics should have much more impact than they have historically. This is a critical distinction from the past, when the metrics deemed most important have been largely operationally or financially oriented (and some would add quality metrics in that mix). For example, as organizations target their audience more definitively, the SL manager will likely be asked to report on ***customer relationship management (CRM)*** campaigns that target—either via traditional mailings or via email campaigns—specific audiences for identified services.

Example CRM metric campaign

One audience-specific CRM campaign might target women ages 25 to 70 for mammography screenings. This kind of CRM approach is a much more measurable way to assess the effectiveness of an outreach campaign and decidedly more accurate in evaluating the cost to benefit or return on investment calculation for the dollars expended for an SL approach. While many healthcare organizations have ramped up CRM efforts in the past several years, CRM campaigns and Web-based outreach are still not as prominent a marketing tactic/approach as in consumer-oriented industries. That will probably change over the next three to five years, as senior executives will demand a greater accuracy and accountability for the dollars expended in the marketing arena.

Marketing will also have a greater say in the cross-sell and "internal capture" functions for services. In a more consumer-driven world, this can be compared to how banks measure their cross-sell effort. For example, Wells Fargo (which some consider the most astute large banking enterprise at cross-selling its services) decided some years ago that it would focus on getting its existing customers to use more of its services, since it is widely known that the effort and expense to have an existing customer add or utilize another service is significantly less than capturing a new customer for that same service.

Consequently, at the time when that strategy was launched, the overall average for services per customer in the banking industry was around 2.5. Within a few years of that declarative strategy and overt attempt at cross-selling services to existing customers, Wells Fargo doubled its average service per customer, reaching more than 5.6 services per customer.

In a hospital setting, CRM can be used to target existing customers/patients for one SL and then cross-sell to a related SL. For example, past patients in the OB/Women's Services SL could receive a mailer for a women's cardiac screening. The data mining abilities exist to determine how many of those women who received the information on the screening were actually screened and then had follow-up services related to the cardiovascular SL. Obviously, this type of specific cross-selling opportunity can and does play out in many instances for various SLs.

Another marketing technique that can fall under the auspices of an astute SL manager is channeling "unaffiliated" patients (i.e., those without a primary care physician, or PCP) from the ER to a PCP within the same system. Some forward-thinking hospitals and health systems have adopted sophisticated Web-based, patient-scheduling systems for onsite assignment of unaffiliated ER patients and schedule the follow-up appointment with a system-affiliated PCP immediately following the individual's ER visit.

This is a win-win situation. The ER patient is connected with a PCP, who can better coordinate his/her ongoing care, and the hospital redirects the ER patient to a more cost-effective care setting, while ensuring that the patient remains within the auspices of the system. Again, electronic databases and Web-based coordination of scheduling have made this process more quantifiable and much more user friendly.

Managing these unaffiliated ER patients becomes even more relevant and beneficial as insurance exchanges/marketplaces are implemented and a wide array of previously uninsured individuals have access to medical care. Many of these newly insured patients will initiate their access to the system via the ER but will not have a PCP. Consequently, hospitals and systems that put measures or protocols into place that assign these people physicians in real time and onsite will provide a service to the patient and retain the individual within their system of care. Along that line, if an organization has ER designated as one of its SLs (and a number of hospitals do), this methodology would actually fall nicely into the business plan and strategy for the ER SL manager.

Quality Measures

As relevant and timely as quantitative metrics have become, organizations will continue to focus on quality measures, such as complication rates or mortality indexes, as these may be driving factors for positioning the organization.

Predictably, such quality measures are becoming a crucial metric for influence-wielding stakeholder groups such as business coalitions or industry entities (e.g., The Leapfrog Group or the Business Roundtable). These metrics have gained a great deal of traction in recent years, and that concentration is likely to intensify over time as employers exhibit more interest and wield more clout in the healthcare arena.

HCAHPS

Hospital Consumer Assessment of Healthcare Providers and Systems (HCAHPS), a national publicly reported data source for quality metrics, has received a great deal of attention from within the industry but not as much attention (as some predicted) from the intended audience—namely, consumers or prospective patients. As a result, HCAHPS use as a reference source has not achieved the level of impact as was originally envisioned.

Still, some predict that awareness of and access to HCAHPS and other quality data will increase significantly as consumers/patients have a greater economic stake in healthcare provider selection and the purchase of services. Even without a significant increase in consumer use of HCAHPS (or other publicly available quality data), including quality measures in your key metrics for SL assessment is a sound strategy for several reasons:

- *First,* it sends a message to all the stakeholder groups that the organization is serious about quality as its *raison d'etre* and committed to monitoring it, comparing it, and enhancing it.

- *Second,* a concerted focus on quality measures is likely to have the desired effect of improving clinical outcomes. In management science, this dynamic often is referred to as the **Hawthorne effect,** which derives its name from an employee study at a Western Electric plant in Hawthorne, Illinois (just outside of Chicago), several decades ago. This managerial phenomenon basically holds that behaviors or indicators that are frequently monitored and measured will often result in improved results, especially within a group setting. In other words, just by shining a bright light on a particular behavior or desired outcome, performance improvement will follow suit. Or, as some have said, improvement comes with measurement.

- *Finally,* given the increased emphasis and scrutiny on quality outcomes, external organizations that showcase and compare standardized quality metrics (like the Leapfrog Group and state data agencies) are getting the jump on provider organizations and—to a certain extent—seizing control of the information reported and reviewed by the public. To that extent, hospital and health system leaders would be wise to get in front of that data reporting movement, or at least embrace it, and align facility goals with publicly reported data.

For these reasons, and given the heightened focus on general transparency throughout the industry (not to mention the impact of accountable care, pay for performance, and other major industry dynamics), you should include at least one quality metric in the five or six main criteria by which the SLs will be identified, arrayed, and prioritized. Practically speaking, if an organization maintains that it is focused squarely on quality but doesn't include quality metrics in the SL performance measure, there is a huge disconnect with the message and the mission of the organization.

Perhaps quality metrics will not achieve the level of awareness and attention that some would hope, but if they do (and I personally believe they will in the next few years), then having a quality metric or two will resonate well with any audience. At present, much of this quality-centered information is being gathered and reported at the broader organizational level, but with the emergence of empowered consumers and population health management, it is only a matter of time until quality metrics cascade down to the SL level. Progressive organizations have already factored such metrics into the overall design and evaluation of SL performance.

Community Need

Another area to consider including in the five or six fundamental metrics by which the organization prioritizes its core SLs is **community need,** or *mission fulfillment*. This metric is consistent with other nonfinancial measures, in that it is more qualitative and also might resonate within some stakeholder circles. A few examples of metrics that could be included in community need include:

- Level of ongoing charity care for the uninsured, even after implementation of insurance exchanges
- Educational efforts centered around health challenges and issues
- Response to specific predominant unmet community needs
- Expenses allocated toward community programs and initiatives as a percentage of net revenue

In recent years, hospitals have been more overt about the level of care they provide to the community that qualifies officially as charity, or what is sometimes called *uncompensated care*. By establishing a metric for the percentage or dollar value of charity care provided and then making that metric public, the hospital or health system educates the community on an important service it provides. For example, some hospitals and health systems include statistics in their annual reports that note something to the effect, "In 2013, St. Anywhere provided over $200 million in charity care and allocated over $50 million in funds to programs that directly affect the community."

Care for the uninsured and the role of exchanges

The issue of uninsured Americans is very much on the minds of most people in the nation, especially with the arrival of insurance exchanges—the cornerstone of the Affordable Care Act (aka Obamacare). Recent surveys show that more individuals now understand and likely appreciate the issue far better than just a few years ago, since the ACA has been such a highly publicized and politically polarizing issue.

Still, some folks do not realize that the exchanges will not eradicate the problem of the uninsured in its entirety. The public likely does have a better appreciation for the fact that the uninsured in America can still get treatment, and that in most cases, the hospitals and health systems bear the financial impact of that problem (at least in a more direct fashion than other players or providers in the system, such as convenient care sites, physician practices, and outpatient surgery centers). Still, most people have no idea as to the extent of this problem and assume that with introduction of insurance exchanges, most of the uninsured will now be covered. Given that perception, some individuals (including politicians) are publicly asking the question, "Do hospitals and other providers—and, in general, the nonprofit sector of healthcare—still deserve their tax exemption?" While the case for eliminating tax exemption for nonprofit entities has not yet reached a fevered pitch (nor even serious broad-based consideration), it will no doubt be raised many times in the next few years, particularly as the ranks of the uninsured diminish appreciably and as providers are reimbursed for the millions of individuals they used to treat for pennies on the dollar or at a fraction of the actual cost.

An interest in preserving future tax exemptions is all the more reason for healthcare providers to track charity care more rigorously and to make a point to publish such statistics broadly. Some states have already established a minimum required percentage of facility revenues that is constituted as "charity care." Those requirements will no doubt get more attention and scrutiny in the years to come. In the next few years, public disclosures of charity care may help to buffer criticism and concern, not only about not-for-profit provider tax exempt status, but also regarding the role that hospitals play in the calculus of increasing prices, a matter of considerable public attention. (Case in point: the *TIME Magazine* March 4, 2013, cover story, "The Bitter Pill: Why Medical Bills are Killing Us.")

All that said, caution should be exercised at the individual market level. Some market research studies have indicated that highlighting the level of charity care provided may not do much for the overall reputation of the hospital and can, in fact, backfire. In some instances, organizations reporting a disproportionately high level of charity care may project the image of a place where only poor people go for treatment. While this resulting perception is indeed an unfortunate conclusion or assumption, I recommend that each organization conduct its own market research to assess the resulting perception when showcasing the level of charity care it provides and the impact on key stakeholders.

The key takeaway in all this is that the measure of charity care and community benefit—much like the quality measures discussed above—should cascade down to the SL level. While not currently tracked or reported at that level in very many organizations, I recommend that such measures be incorporated into the ongoing performance assessment of the core SLs. As the public becomes more aware and engaged in the purchase and provision of healthcare, they will want that level of transparency and will appreciate the reporting and relevance of such measures at the consumer-facing level.

To determine how to communicate about charity care, organizations should survey their own stakeholders to gauge the effect of such messaging. This is especially true in the wake of the changes that have occurred due to the Affordable Care Act (ACA). The issue of undocumented individuals will continue to loom large in this area and will be a matter that each community will wrestle with post-ACA implementation.

Educational efforts

Healthcare institutions can be invaluable vehicles for communication when it comes to local health-related issues. Some hospitals have established goals in terms of communicating in their community the effects of serious illnesses that are to some extent related to lifestyle. Some examples include obesity, diabetes, certain cancers, heart disease, and so forth.

As the acknowledged hub of the healthcare sector, hospitals and health systems lend both credence and clout to messages about health issues. They also are arguably in the best position to coordinate such messaging in concert with associations (such as the American Heart Association, the American Diabetes Association, the American Lung Association, and so forth), community groups, employers, and other interested parties.

Some hospitals and health systems still have education departments (although the number has diminished with cost-cutting efforts throughout the industry), so it is possible to incorporate educational campaigns and initiatives. And, like the ongoing uncompensated care issue, health and fitness concerns are emerging as a much more relevant and timely consideration as the focus shifts to population health and to the provider's responsibility in not just treating sick people but monitoring and maintaining (and being reimbursed for) the overall well-being of a defined population.

Once the dust settles on exchanges and the implementation of the ACA, the matter of population health, and the pivotal role of providers in orchestrating that movement, will receive much media attention and public concern. For example, what role will hospitals and physicians play in addressing and mitigating the rising problem of obesity, which is identified as a greater health concern than smoking? Hospitals or health systems that lead the charge in an educational and assistance campaign on obesity will not only glean a great deal of favorable publicity but will also perform a valuable service to the community.

While on the subject of exchanges, many hospitals and systems throughout the country took a key role (either on their own or in partnership with organizations such as Enroll America) in enrolling insurance exchange participants. Some provider systems, like Trinity Health (now CHE Trinity), headquartered in Livonia, Michigan, choreographed extensive ground campaigns to inform the public about the basic elements of exchanges and then to enroll as many people as they could in their associated communities throughout the nation.

Trinity's large-scale, effectively coordinated effort had at its core a direct link to the organization's mission to provide care in the communities in which the system was located and, as part of that mission, to increase access to care for the uninsured and underinsured. The organization's high-profile effort involved hundreds of individuals within the organization, from the community benefit function to the patient financial services department.

This type of educational initiative and community outreach effort pays dividends for any provider organization, and in a more consumer-driven world, it engenders not only community good will but also ongoing patient/consumer loyalty. As we look toward the future, such community outreach and educational efforts can be effectively choreographed at an SL level. Many of these campaigns and initiatives center around a specific disease category or health issue (e.g., obesity, cardiovascular disease, cancer-related illnesses, etc.), and so it makes perfect sense to have the SL leaders and their matrix teams lead out with these initiatives.

Response to unmet needs

Many health systems focus on those areas of the business or the field that provide a meaningful and sustainable return on their investment. That is natural and in most cases appropriate. Yet there are some unmet needs within the community that may never provide such a financial return.

Encompassed in most healthcare organizations' mission is the desire to improve the overall health of the community. By establishing a metric that incorporates the general well-being of the community (or in broader strokes, humanity), the hospital or health system is communicating that profit isn't everything, or even the most important thing. Fundamentally meeting the needs of the community is.

Some skeptics may scoff at this type of reasoning, but healthcare leaders need to recognize the perceptual corner into which we have been boxed. As one savvy investment analyst noted some years back, "There is still a negative perception in the public around the idea of organizations and individuals getting rich off the backs of sick people."

Despite evidence to the contrary, the abiding perception is that hospitals are highly profitable enterprises. Even though most people who work within the industry know that the average NOI calculation is around 3% for hospitals across the country, research demonstrates that the public either doesn't know or doesn't want to believe that fact.

Consequently, including metrics like community need helps diffuse the misperception that hospitals are interested in profit before patients, and it helps instill in the public's mind the notion that hospitals really are about caring, not just cash. More importantly, as with the charity care and education, it brings the organizations (at least the nonprofit enterprises) back to their reason for being, which really *is* to enhance the healthcare of the community.

Core Metric Performance by SL

From the broad categories listed above, an organization should focus on the four or five measures that matter most to the key stakeholder groups. These can be presented in a number of different formats, but I recommend using some form of two-dimension table, as it provides an easy-to-understand graphic snapshot. This rather simple graphic can also be shared with various key stakeholder groups, including the board of directors and community partners.

Figure 7.1| Dual-axis matrix representation of SLs by metrics

Core Organization Metrics: Performance by Service Line				
	Orthopedics	Oncology	Cardiology CV	General Surgery	Enterprise All SLs
Net Operating Income %	15%	6%	22%	18%	5%
Market Share %	35%	28%	31%	42%	38%
Quality Ranking	75th percentile	68th percentile	70th percentile	85th percentile	72nd percentile
Charity Care %	5%	10%	4%	6%	7%
Community Outreach	Medium	High	Low	Medium	Medium

Figure 7.1 shows what one nonprofit community hospital chose as the five salient criteria (or metrics) for assessing the performance of their SLs:

- NOI for the entire SL

- Market share relative to competition in the area

- Percentile ranking for complications vis à vis national averages

- Percentile ranking for mortality vis à vis national averages

- Percentage of charity care provided for that SL

- Opportunities/performance in fulfilling community needs and outreach within that SL

Once the data for these metrics have been gathered for all the SLs, they then can be arrayed by category, within each core SL.

For the financial measures and even the quality metrics or indices, the critical lines will stand out rather readily (for many facilities, cardiology/CV, orthopedics, oncology, and general surgery). The other metrics (e.g., community need or outreach) may be more difficult to assess and to measure, but that should not prohibit these metrics from being part of the overall performance scorecard.

The ranking mechanism or formula used will depend on the goals, philosophy, and strategic direction/orientation of each organization. The key is that by diversifying the measures a bit (so that not only financial and volume measures are included), the organization is sending an important message that there is more to success than merely meeting or exceeding the bottom line and that hospitals are in the business of caring and are not just focused on caring about the business.

Faith in market-driven metrics

As noted earlier, with the expected shift to more of a consumer-driven environment, your list of key organizational measures should be updated to incorporate more market-driven metrics in gauging the effectiveness of your SL performance.

A case in point is a recent decision by a large faith-based system headquartered in the Southwest to pare its **core strategic marketing metrics** to these five (out of a total of 21 that were identified by the SL leaders and marketing directors):

1. Market share (both inpatient and outpatient against the key competitor)

2. Website visits

3. Monthly visits by the physician liaisons to the doctors in the primary service area

4. Contribution margin on CRM campaigns

5. Volume increase attributed to cross-sell initiatives by SL

Conclusion

Whatever measures are selected as most important for the organization's long-term viability and competitive position in the market, the lesson here is that early identification of what matters most will assist all those who are being held accountable for the success of the individual SLs. Additionally, the metric identification, followed by the core SL selection, allows the organization to deploy its resources in the areas that are most essential for long-term viability.

By identifying these mission-essential metrics, senior leadership empowers the management team to concentrate their time and attention on the things that matter most, an invaluable advantage in times of flux and increasing consumer-driven market dynamics.

8

Identifying the Core Service Lines

Getting to the Core

Once you've completed the difficult work of defining the framework for your service lines (SL), (e.g., diagnosis-related groups [DRG], International Classification of Diseases [ICD], etc.) and have determined the key organizational metrics for assessing the success of each, it's time to identify the core lines.

Identifying the few SLs that are essential to the organization's success is not as easy as it may sound. You will undoubtedly meet resistance when you select the primary, focused group of SLs that will (at least initially) receive disproportionate resources and managerial attention. Nonetheless, it is a process that must occur, as it does in most successful organizations in other industries and among progressive enterprises in our field.

Portfolio analysis

One of the most effective methods for prioritization is to conduct a ***portfolio analysis***—that is, a process by which you create an array of the SLs and then rank them based on the metrics established by each related group, as discussed previously in Chapters 5 and 7. This internal assessment is an important step in helping the hospital or health system identify the SLs that constitute the bulk of the firm's revenue, profitability, patient volume, or whatever key metrics the organization has identified. These criteria for prioritizing the key SLs should reflect the organization's competitive market position, and their selection as the "core few" should also resonate with the key stakeholder groups, patients, consumers, and physicians.

Though you can expect that prioritizing the organization's SLs may engender a certain degree of executive angst, you will create a more nimble organization prepared to face an increasingly competitive field. In fact, if you got only this far in the SL process, namely the identification and agreement on the core SLs/business units, the ensuing results would make the entire effort worthwhile.

The Pareto Principle applied to hospital strategy

In essence, the prioritization that takes place with the SL model is nothing more than a data-driven implementation of the Pareto Principle, which we discussed earlier in the book.

Vilfredo Pareto was an Italian economist and Renaissance man who believed that roughly 20% of an entity's effort would produce approximately 80% of its key results or outcomes. For hospitals or health systems, those key results (the 80%) include net revenue, contribution margin (CM), or operating income/profitability.

The secret to successfully employing Pareto analysis is to correctly identify the most productive 20% (or thereabouts) and then be willing to concentrate the organization's planning and resources on those high-performing segments of the overall operation.

Practical application of two-dimension graphics

Earlier, we discussed how the organization must identify the metrics that define its success. These metrics include the standard measurements of organizational effectiveness and long-term viability, such as net revenue, CM and market share or growth potential. These three measurements, and others you may chose, can be displayed graphically to demonstrate the relative strength of the organization's SLs.

Let's look at how this was done for one particular hospital in the Southwest. The graph in Figure 8.1 is one form of illustration for a *portfolio analysis,* and it depicts all of the hospital's SLs with two dimensions in consideration, discharges by category or SL and contribution margin per discharge for each of the SLs identified.

Figure 8.1| Service line Pareto analysis chart

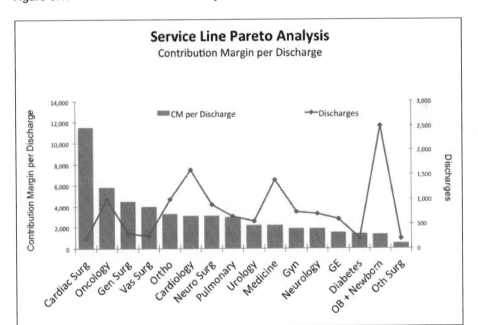

This type of depiction or portfolio analysis can be used to select the four or five SLs that will constitute the core SLs identified for the SL structure employed by designated SL managers/directors, matrix teams, business plans, etc. In our example, if senior leadership at the hospital determines that CM per discharge is the driving factor in selecting the core SLs, then those five, certainly the top four (and perhaps orthopedics), will receive most of the organization's time, effort, and resources, such as capital expenditures, upgraded equipment, and marketing dollars.

What you see in Figure 8.1 is a good example of the Pareto Principle in application, as the five SLs on the left side of the chart (cardiac surgery, oncology, general surgery, vascular surgery, and orthopedics) represent about 20% of the total discharges but 64% of the CM per discharge for this hospital. The graph clearly indicates that the hospital should emphasize SLs such as cardiac surgery and oncology because of their higher-than-average CM per discharge and, to a lesser extent, general surgery and vascular surgery.

After the first four SLs, the CM per discharge drops off rather sharply. However, the other dimension of this graphic is the discharges per SL, and for this organization, even though cardiac surgery has a very high CM per discharge, the category has a small number of discharges (less than 1,000). On the other hand, of the top five SLs, oncology and orthopedics have high total discharges, which means that the total CM for those SLs would be quite high and may be reason enough to consider designating orthopedics as one of the core SLs.

Along that line, the same can be said for cardiology, which is sixth in terms of CM per discharge but has the second highest number of discharges in this organization, again equating to a high total CM. Given this picture, the organization may choose to combine cardiac surgery, vascular surgery, and cardiology into one strategic business unit, the cardiovascular (CV) SL, and by so doing, narrow the top six SLs (as arrayed by CM per discharge) into four; CV, oncology, general surgery, and orthopedics. By selecting these SLs as the core, the organization captures the six top CM per discharge areas, which account for more than 60% of the total CM as well.

On the other end of the spectrum, as this chart indicates, the SL with the highest number of discharges is OB + newborn, which has nearly twice as many discharges as the second-highest volume SL, but has the second-lowest CM per discharge (only other surgery is lower) for all the SLs measured. As mentioned earlier in the book, this type of analysis not only highlights the SLs worth emphasizing, it can also illuminate those that might be candidates for "demarketing" or consolidation, or elimination altogether. This kind of relative financial positioning assessment has led more than a few hospitals and health systems to drop OB services at their facilities or at least to scale back on their efforts in that segment of the business for that very reason.

A word of caution about assumptions

As basic as this kind of analysis may seem, the fact remains that in many healthcare organizations, the leading SLs—those that are absolutely critical to the hospital or health system's success—do not receive attention commensurate with their contribution to the overall success of the enterprise. In fact, since these lines have proven to be so successful over time, there is a counterproductive tendency to regard them as "slam dunks" and therefore to concentrate on other areas or services that represent future revenue streams or margin opportunities.

Assuming ongoing success for leading SLs is a precarious strategy that has not played out well in many markets and for numerous organizations. For example, in years past, many hospitals did not commit the time and resources to the high-margin business units such as cardiology. Too late, they realized their folly, as specialty hospitals, niche players, or physician-led initiatives drained off their business and eroded their revenue streams and higher margins. More recently, changes in reimbursement and classification for cardiac procedures have eroded the overall financial contribution of this heretofore leading-performance SL. Firms such as the Advisory Board and Sg2 forecast that such economic diminution in the cardiac SL will continue in the next few years.

Unfortunately, there is no guarantee that a concerted emphasis on a particular SL will either stave off competitive forces or mitigate diminishing reimbursement, but focused attention and keen awareness of the market dynamics and external influences can definitely provide greater intelligence and a better understanding and appreciation of what lies on the horizon.

In many cases, if more attention had been paid to key physicians and core services in those profitable SLs rather than assuming self-sustaining success, the organization may have been able to create its own center of excellence or medical service arena with regional drawing power and increased market differentiation, alleviating physician exodus, discouraging new competitors, and avoiding the ensuing decline in volume that further erodes the strength of the overall SL.

Shifting Away from the Traditional 'Core Four' SLs

We know that one reason the landscape is changing for the traditional core SLs is the move by the Centers for Medicare & Medicaid Services (CMS) to recalibrate the reimbursement framework and payment structure. For planning purposes, organizations must reconsider the degree to which their organization can rely on their traditional core SLs. In addition, they must conduct sophisticated scenario-planning exercises that factor in the newly reconfigured payment algorithms.

All this does not mean that hospitals should abandon their current strategies with these high-margin SLs, as the new reimbursement configurations may not shift the reimbursement architecture as dramatically as some have predicted. It will, however, have financial impact on organizations that derive a great deal of their total volume from surgical procedures, especially in cardiology.

The impact of reimbursement on SL framework

Organizations should adjust not only their financial projections but their marketing and advertising budgets and strategies to offset the effects of the latest CMS reimbursement adjustments. The revised payment structure has already begun to alter the basic framework of an SL's traditional standing. For example, in recent years, many CV procedures have moved from an inpatient (IP) setting to an outpatient (OP) venue.

In the period since the introduction of the inpatient prospective payment system, the healthcare industry has experienced a dramatic reduction in the volume of IP cases in the CV SL, and a similar uptick in OP volumes. Unfortunately, conversion to the OP classification has produced sharp reductions in net revenue, as the reimbursement for the OP classification is markedly lower than for the prior IP categorization.

Many providers have seen a significant drop in CV net revenue and net operating income (NOI), as well as a noticeable decline in the percentage of CV SL revenue and NOI. The downward trend is expected to continue in CV and other high-margin SLs, due to both CMS and private payer strategies to move high-cost procedures into more efficient, less expensive venues. Recent reclassification and accompanying reimbursement trends reflect that cost-saving shift.

In addition to factoring in modifications to the reimbursement model, it goes without saying that every organization, and especially SL leaders, will also need to monitor the federal legislation and regulation related to specialty hospitals and physician investment in hospitals and other healthcare institutions. Federal regulations have already had and could continue to have a rather dramatic effect on specialty services, even if such legislation effectively grandfathers existing niche players or specialty hospitals, allowing them to continue to provide physician ownership, or what is sometimes referred to as syndication.

Sponsoring organizations, such as private-equity firms or Wall Street companies, may be reluctant to invest much money in a model that has limited long-term growth prospects. As much as anything, these market dynamics are being influenced by the move to physician employment by hospitals and health systems nationwide. The number of employed physicians has skyrocketed over the last five to 10 years and shows no signs of abatement. There are a number of reasons for the growth of this strategy, not the least of which is the ability of the sponsoring organization (hospital or health system) to effectively solidify the referral patterns of the employed physicians.

The staff model has also proven its worth in the context of population health management. Those systems touted as the most efficient and effective in managing defined populations and controlling utilization (including the marquee players; Mayo Clinic, Cleveland Clinic, Geisinger, Scott & White, Intermountain Health Care and Kaiser) all employ staff models. Pluralistic systems—those with a combination of employed physicians and independent doctors—are in essence trying to move to a model for population health management, and, in so doing, many are acquiring as many physicians as they can.

To that end, this trend of health systems purchasing niche players—or *focused factories,* as they are sometimes called—has modified somewhat in recent years. In many instances, when a health system considers the purchase of a large physician practice, any enterprise in which the physicians have invested (e.g., specialty hospital, imaging center, and so forth) is a major part of the deal and comes along with the purchase. As a result, larger health systems that don't already have a few niche players in their portfolio, either as wholly owned entities or comanaged and/or coowned entities, are the exception rather than the norm.

And even more telling in these days of creative arrangements and portfolio expansion is the trend of large systems to include a new breed of enterprise in the overall portfolio. In addition to horizontal mergers and acquisitions or affiliations (hospital with hospital, health system with health system) and vertical combinations (hospital with physician practices) are what could be termed "diagonal" arrangements or acquisitions. These diagonal acquisitions involve health-related enterprises that have potential for synergy or symbiosis but not in the traditional view of M&A activity. Examples of these new arrangements are Dignity's purchase of U.S. HealthWorks, Tenet's ownership in Conifer, and one of the original such ventures, Ascension's involvement with Accretive Health.

Using portfolio analysis in a more complex fashion

All that noted, you are probably wondering, what does the more traditional portfolio analysis process look like? Figure 8.2 depicts a graphic that is used in many portfolio assessments and is sometimes referred to as a "bubble chart." The difference between this approach and the two-factor chart referenced earlier is that this provides a more expansive view of the SLs and uses three dimensions to array the SLs. In this revealing snapshot of the organization, the three dimensions, or performance measures of each SL are market share (shown on the Y axis), projected SL growth rate (shown on the X axis) and CM per case (relative size of the bubble).

Figure 8.2 | Portfolio assessment bubble chart

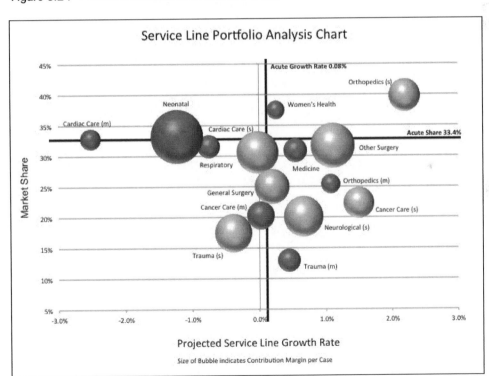

Unlike Figure 8.1, which analyzed only the relative financial strength of each SL, this graphic includes the competitive position for each business unit—both current and projected. By taking into consideration these other two dimensions or performance criteria, the organization is able to consider the value of the SL in a more strategic capacity.

For example, in the case of this organization, the orthopedics SL has both the highest market share of all the SLs and the highest projected growth rate over the next 3–5 years. While the ortho SL does not have the highest CM per case or discharge (it is actually sixth in that category), it ranks higher than many of the other SLs.

In terms of CM/case, the neonatal segment of the business has clearly the highest performance in that category, but it is right on the organizational average in terms of market share and has the second-lowest projected growth rate (second only to medical cardiac care) in the next few years. This graphic also differentiates between medical and procedural (primarily surgery) cases. As depicted in the chart, and as is the situation with most hospitals and health systems, the procedural areas of the enterprise have considerably higher margins per case than do the medical.

Weighing all three factors—market share, growth rate, and CM/case—this organization's major investment in SL development and growth appears to lie in the northeast quadrant of the chart, with orthopedics (surgery), other surgery, and women's health the likely candidates for managerial attention and resource allocation, if factoring in growth rate and market share; and for neonatal, cardiac care (surgery), neurological (surgery) and trauma (surgery) if the focus is on CM/case.

The analysis reflected above is yet another way to assess the relative strength of the SLs but may not be the only gauge or picture to view. Another important managerial exercise is to take several different snapshots of the organization. The chart in Figure 8.2 provides market-competitive and growth potential assessments as well, which are highly important in the overall evaluation. Progressive organizations will consider and develop a number of analyses and market measurements that provide a variety of scenarios. Each scenario slices the data differently, thus allowing you to consider several different variables as you work to determine your core SLs. For example, the criteria that have been presented in the aforementioned graphs are primarily financial—with some consideration for market growth. Yet there obviously are several other relevant and essential criteria to consider.

These criteria could include ensuring access, providing services, accomplishing missions, aligning with physician interests, and so forth. Some of these determinants are more readily quantified than others and thus more easily graphed. The more qualitative variables can be assigned numerical values based on consensus of key stakeholders or stakeholder groups—or based on the assessment of senior management.

Whatever technique is employed, the fact remains that most—if not all—criteria for assigning and ranking organizational value can and should be quantified and depicted in readily understood graphics.

In truth, most organizations in these times will use criteria that are financially oriented or market growth/share-based, or a combination of those two. However, that does not preclude any organization from also factoring in criteria of mission fulfillment or community need, as discussed in Chapter 7. These criteria will prove to be important, especially for nonprofit governance bodies (such as the board of trustees). These types of criteria also should be considered in light of other key stakeholder groups, such as community leaders, donors, politicians, and even the media.

At the very least, conducting quality-based analysis that factors in variables other than economic, growth potential, and market share measures will demonstrate that the organization considers other essential variables in assessing which lines matter most. Such analysis also will prove valuable when it comes time for the organization to decide which SLs should be consolidated, shifted to another provider or delivery source, or eliminated altogether. For example, as noted above, even though a fair number of hospitals have decided to eliminate obstetrics from their portfolio, other organizations have chosen to retain those services due to community need (no other close-proximity provider), even though economically that SL was not a significant contributor.

In making those decisions, the organization's aims are quite different: It must focus on reasons why a line should be allocated time and resources (or exist at all), rather than just focusing on the lines that matter most. If the organization has factored in key evaluation criteria for the leading SLs at the outset, then the leaders of the enterprise will be both more comfortable with the exercise and adept at its implementation.

Conclusion

In these times of limited capital and unlimited need, one of the most important things an organization can do is identify and then communicate the areas of operation that matter most to the long-term viability of the enterprise. Proactive service line management (SLM) offers a framework that can help identify the core areas of the entity's operation (i.e., those that constitute the economic essence of the organization and account for the lion's share of its financial stability).

By using the criteria for evaluation discussed previously in the book, senior management can highlight those core lines (no more than three or four at the outset) that offer the best potential for growth and, at the same time, offer the greatest contribution to the bottom line. These factors of financial strength and market potential are likely to be the driving criteria for selecting the core SLs, but the organization also can factor in qualitative considerations such as community benefit, mission fulfillment, or perceived stakeholder value.

Whatever the criteria chosen for identifying the "core few" and then paring down the SLs to a manageable number, this exercise enables management to concentrate its resources and attention on critical services that represent the leading source of financial stability. These key SLs face numerous competitive market forces, ranging from physician ventures to emerging competition. A focused SL effort is one of the best structures for shoring up the base, as well as for fending off the competition.

Organizing for
Market Orientation
and Consumer/Patient
Proximity

Once you've identified and communicated your short list of core service lines (SL), it's time to establish the optimal managerial structure. As for so many of the fundamental building blocks of service line management (SLM), defining the correct managerial structure for your organization is challenging; there is no one-size-fits-all formula for success. Some structures work better than others, due to the nature of the model and the requirements of the job. A number of preferred and highly successful structures have emerged from industries outside healthcare, including one I recommend most often and will describe in depth in this chapter: a matrix managerial structure that involves a variety of functions and individuals.

All that said, when people ask which organizational structure works best, the safest and most accurate answer is, "The one that matches your market."

Getting Started

Although you'll find no shortage of approaches to managing SLs, you'll want to consider time-tested approaches that have been shown to deliver the basic elements of a successful structure. You'll also want to evaluate potential designs for a few key components.

First, it's essential for long-term success that you incorporate sufficient **authority** and **accountability** within the chosen management design. Without accountability and authority, the overall model will hobble along and achieve moderate results at best. I've observed organizations where there is ample responsibility but insufficient authority—those models have usually produced suboptimal outcomes.

As Groucho Marx famously quipped, "The two most important things in life are honesty and sincerity. If you can fake those, you've got it made." In the case of successful SLM, the organization cannot fake accountability and authority.

Although there is variation between successful models, there are some common elements and measurements that can be applied across operational structures. With that in mind, consider the following proven models.

The Matrix Model

When the concept of SLM was new to the field, one of the most popular models for organizational design was a **matrix construct**. Unlike a direct-line authority model, where everyone under the auspices of the manager or director reports directly to him or her, under a matrix model, the SL manager is responsible for a team, but most, if not all, of those individuals don't report to him or her. In essence, under a matrix model, the SL manager relies on informal authority, and the other members of the team are often at a peer level or higher. Adopted from organizations such as Procter & Gamble and other consumer goods enterprises, this model had been tested and proven over decades of successful application.

The value of the matrix model is that it spreads the responsibility across several functions and departments and thus encourages both input and ownership throughout the organization. This construct was particularly valuable in the early days of product line management (or SLM), when the concept needed to gain broad-scale awareness and organizationwide acceptance. To that end, the matrix design still should be considered a viable option for SL managerial architecture. This is especially true in organizations that are not familiar with the SL structure.

Admittedly, there are at least two downsides to a matrix orientation, however. First, as noted earlier, healthcare administration tends to be rather traditional and thus hierarchical. Healthcare administration follows the military model, which is as close to the antithesis of matrix management as a management style can get.

Figure 9.1| A service line matrix model

Service Line Management Matrix by Function								
	Finance	Physician Advisor	Marketing-PR	Exec. Team	Lab	Diag.	Supply-Chain	Coding
Cardiovascular *SL Manager*								
Orthopedics *SL Manager*								
Neurosciences *SL Manager*								
Oncology *SL Manager*								
Gen. Surgery *SL Manager*								

Many healthcare executives may be uncomfortable with matrix management: It requires not only a new mind-set but also a different reporting and accountability structure. There are a fair number of senior executives in healthcare who say, "I want to have one person ultimately responsible." Although that dynamic still is possible under a matrix design, the input measurement and feedback cycles are different than under the traditional structure.

The second downside—which can also be an upside—is that it spreads the accountability, which can be similarly uncomfortable or foreign to the long-standing managerial architecture. Yet this approach has been proven to be highly effective not only in consumer goods organizations but also in leading managerial models. The team product launch and product management are core ideas to emerge from the Deming approach and other quality improvement applications. This concept is often cited as a driver of enhanced quality and so-called "owned" responsibility, because it involves a wider array of functions within the organization. It is also viewed as more "peer to peer," and thus both the awareness of the product or service initiative, as well as its ultimate success, are viewed as a team effort, in the truest sense of that dynamic.

While the matrix design may not be the standard approach in healthcare management, the very nature of the care delivery model is, in fact, multifaceted and collaborative. An individual entering a hospital interacts with a variety of functions, crossing departmental boundaries and requiring considerable coordination. It follows then that a matrix-style planning and strategy execution team would be effective in optimizing the success of an SL, provided they have the buy-in to do so.

In practice, individuals involved in the delivery of care or other facets of interaction with an SL will eventually become involved with that particular line at some point in time. Involving them at the outset guarantees their contribution early on and throughout the process and enhances their ownership in the ongoing success of that particular line.

The optimal matrix team manager

Predictably, the core member of the matrix team is the **SL manager or director**. This role is critical to any organizational design; the fundamental managerial requirements do not change materially depending on the organizational model. However, under a matrix organization, more consideration should be given to the scope of the position and thus to the individual who fills it.

In an organization employing a matrix structure, the SL director needs to be an astute *influence* or informal manager. That is not a skill set that all managers possess, especially if they have practiced most of their career under a line authority model. Influence management requires the ability to persuade more than mandate, relying on interpersonal skills more than on derived or stated authority.

Based on my observation, a dedicated SL manager is the key ingredient for any configuration. If the organization can institute an organizational structure of capable and *dedicated* SL managers, it is likely to experience greater success. By dedicated, I mean SL managers are focused on the management of their SLs and are not wearing that hat along with other hats related to managerial responsibility. Additionally, they are not responsible for the management of multiple SLs.

There are two reasons that managers responsible only for their SL are more likely to succeed. First, the SL manager is able to concentrate his or her complete attention on one particular SL. In contrast, senior managers, department directors, or assistant administrators who assume the responsibility for an SL along with their other duties will almost always be pulled back to their preexisting responsibilities. Someone with a singular focus is more likely to succeed than someone who is being asked to multitask.

The second reason has as much to do with the organizational dynamic and perception as the individual's focus or ability. Assigning a dedicated manager sends a strong message and communicates the significant value assigned to that SL—and the overall strategic emphasis placed on the SL approach. If the responsibility for a high-profile SL is given to a current manager as an add-on responsibility, the perceived commitment to the overall SL approach and to the specific SL will be devalued, if not compromised. There is a certain organizational cachet in singular focus, and much greater recognition and empowerment in dedicated responsibility.

Admittedly, not all organizations can afford dedicated SL managers for each of their SLs. Harking back to the inherent value of the Pareto analysis, however, if an organization carefully and thoughtfully defines and outlines the organizational value of its three or four core SLs, executives will quickly recognize that devoting one individual—even if he or she is highly compensated—to the cardiology or cardiovascular SL, for example, is a relatively small investment to ensure sizeable revenue retention.

It really boils down to the "aha factor," which is why the first few steps of arraying the SLs and highlighting the relative impact or significance of the top three or four will make it easier to allocate resources to those critical service areas. For example, one 400-bed hospital decided to ramp up its cardiovascular (CV) SL, recognizing the value of that strategic business unit to the organization. The hospital hired a seasoned clinical manager with established business acumen and committed significant resources to the CV line. The investment paid off handsomely: The organization established a center of excellence for that service, dramatically increased referrals to the specialists, experienced a marked increase in volume and revenue, and created a valuable template for the other core SLs in its portfolio.

Stated another way, compensation on the order of $80,000 to $160,000 to effectively and successfully manage a business unit that generates tens of millions of dollars in net revenue and several million dollars in NOI seems like a reasonable investment.

Sample job description for SL manager or director

The SL manager is responsible for management, development, financial control, measurement, and implementation of program initiatives for clinical service at *St. Anywhere*. The right person for this role will be familiar with hospital operations, will be familiar with the language and roles of this particular service, and will facilitate communication and relations with physicians, hospital leadership, and other key stakeholders.

This role requires skills in project management, marketing and strategic planning, team building, negotiation, business management, and analysis. In addition, candidates will be expected to demonstrate success in generating volume growth for an assigned SL as well as the ability to create and implement strategies for its development, including the geographic market and the interrelationship with the other key services at *St. Anywhere*.

Minimum qualifications include:

1. Bachelor's degree in business, healthcare, or related field; master's degree preferred in business, healthcare, or related field.

2. Eight to 10 years of professional experience in hospital operations and/or consulting (significant documented track record of success and/or graduate degree may be considered as a substitute for years of professional work experience).

3. Excellent verbal, written, budgeting, analytical, time management, and interpersonal skills. Candidates must be able to manage large projects, measure results, and both establish and meet deadlines.

4. Proficiency with Microsoft Office, including Excel, PowerPoint, and other related products. Additional knowledge and expertise of software and information systems related to this service are preferred. Social media acumen is required.

5. The ability to perform duties in a manner that promotes quality patient care and adheres to the mission, vision, and values of *St. Anywhere*.

Finding consumer-savvy SL leaders

Of course, the bigger challenge as our industry adjusts a shifting market landscape and newly engaged consumers is to find managers or directors who understand consumer-facing dynamics and who can transition from the traditional managerial model. To be successful, SL managers must fully understand the dramatic changes in the way care will be accessed and reimbursement will be realized.

To that end, organizations should seriously consider employing one or two individuals in SL leadership with experience in other consumer-facing industries. This resource pool could also include professionals who have worked in the more consumer-facing facets of healthcare, such as the pharmaceutical industry, or even the insurance sector. These people have experience dealing with a retail market dynamic, from promotion to individual-payment interaction. Marketing professionals from packaged goods or highly promotion-centric industries are also good candidates.

One of the main reasons for tapping into expertise from market-facing industries is the ability to engage and communicate effectively with individuals via social media, blogging, email, and the like and to fully understand and appreciate the power of social networks. This is where the game has shifted in our day.

Healthcare will experience significant and disruptive changes from the impact of the digital overlay because, as an industry, it is currently so far behind in implementing digital access, information-sharing, and transaction orientation. Consequently, most healthcare managers and executives will be unprepared for the full impact of communication networks on traditional hierarchical management structure and approach.

My advice? Hire a few seasoned new media/social media veterans (although they'll likely be younger than anyone else on the management team) to navigate the uncharted waters of digital transformation.

The rest of the matrix team

Once a manager is hired, he or she can be instrumental in identifying the remaining members of the matrix team. There are no standard selection criteria, but the list below identifies some of the functions to consider, including:

- Finance
- Marketing or public relations
- Clinical leadership or nursing

- Web expert (social media and Internet communication)

- Lab

- Medical advisor (physician in that area)

- Ancillary functions (where applicable)

- Diagnostic area

- Coding or billing (if the financial member doesn't represent those functions)

- Senior management or administration (vice president or equivalent)

- Materials management

- Other functions or departments that have high involvement in that particular SL

Although it's by no means comprehensive, this list represents the type of individuals and functions that should be part of the team and that will contribute to the overall success of the SL

Clinical Design with Adjunct Committee Structure

Unlike a matrix design, a clinical design more closely follows a traditional hospital organization style, which may make it easier to implement. Most hospitals work within an established department head structure, and a clinical SL design involves working within a similar framework that has been augmented to include other departments.

Incorporating these other functional areas (e.g., finance, marketing, materials management/supply chain, etc.) is essential within the SL planning and implementation design. By not including a variety of functional areas or related departments, the organization has done little more than put a new name on an old design. As provincial as this may sound, some organizations have done just that, thinking (somehow) that by adding the moniker of SLM, they will modify the structure and change the outcome. (Good luck with that.)

To be successful, you must refine the organizational design as well as the market orientation of the new structure. Your new SL design will incorporate the authority and accountability mentioned at the outset of this chapter and extend them to the key functions within the organization.

System Structure for Consumer Alignment

So what is the best configuration for managing SLs within a health system with several facilities? The answer depends on the system's model and strategic orientation.

If the system is pursuing a **clinical center of excellence** approach, where it focuses its efforts and resources on one flagship facility or campus, then it probably is best to centralize the SLM responsibilities at the system level. If, on the other hand, the system is intent on developing the SLs at each facility with little in common among those lines (perhaps other than marketing and contractor), then it is likely best to use a **decentralized structure**, with SL responsibility located at each of the facilities.

There are several reasons for this approach. **First**, getting close to the customer and anticipating the needs of the market is difficult to do on a regional or mult-isystem level because, as we know, all healthcare is local. Having one SL manager for multiple facilities in diverse markets diminishes your ability to engage the key customers (especially physicians). This would be especially problematic in markets where physicians are considering or already pursuing entrepreneurial ventures. In these cases, it's essential to be able to anticipate the needs of the market and to preempt the emerging competition.

The other reason to use a decentralized structure lies in the nature of the organization. As emphasized throughout this chapter, there is great value in getting the input and involvement of many different individuals and stakeholder groups within and throughout the organization. This is difficult to do at the system level, as things tend to become too general and theoretical. It is better to operate and analyze at the level where the customers are interacting, which is within the facility. The reality is that patients usually don't relate to cardiology services across a system. Rather, they relate to how cardiac care is delivered at a particular hospital with a specific doctor and an individualized team of caregivers.

I have seen models where multihospital systems—especially in tighter geographic regions—have utilized a senior SL director who oversees the work and output of the SL managers/directors at the other facilities. For example, a three-hospital system in southern New Jersey employed just such a model; they had SL directors for oncology at each of the hospitals, but one of those directors had ultimate responsibility and accountability for the performance of the oncology SL across the system. The other two SL directors had dual reporting relationships to their CEO and to the senior director. That model worked well for that system, and in that particular SL.

Every organization is different, and what works for one hospital or health system may not work for another. But based on my experiences with many different hospitals, a multifunctional SL team functioning in a matrix model, with the SL manager as the leader of the team, is usually the most effective, as I stated at the outset of the chapter.

Conclusion

As time and experience have shown me, the caliber of leadership most often determines the ultimate success of an enterprise or an endeavor. SLM is no different. Unfortunately, too many organizations do not devote enough consideration to the issue of managing or leading the SL construct. And that is often the point at which the SL implementation slouches toward mediocrity.

To avoid that unfortunate and unnecessary outcome, your senior leaders should keep a few key things in mind as they institute the SL model. First, select a qualified SL manager or director, one with not only the technical savvy to lead the effort, but the interpersonal ability to direct a team effort. Second, I recommend a multidisciplinary matrix team that involves key individuals and departments that naturally interact with the SL and have a stake in its ultimate success. Finally, senior leadership needs to remain integrally involved in the design, development, monitoring, and ongoing reassessment and recalibration of the SL team effort. If the senior executive team is committed to SL success and demonstrates serious commitment with its time, involvement, and resource allocation, that will go a long way in ensuring the success of the SL model.

10

Assessing Perception and Market Position by Service Line

Over the past five to 10 years, some of the largest and most consumer-savvy organizations in the nation have recognized the economic and market potential of the healthcare provider space. You know them as household names: Walmart, Target, CVS, Walgreens, etc. To date, a large number of healthcare executives have inexplicably ignored (and continue to ignore) the competitive threat of these new entrants into the market.

Healthcare executives who aren't yet concerned about this raft of competitors need a serious dose of reality. Those unquestioning executives fail to grasp the implications of the retail giants' play for our business. Some executives have discounted the threat of big-box competitors because of a provincial focus on traditional competitors. Others have felt that the newcomers would fade away or at least not encroach significantly on the legacy business.

Both assumptions were incorrect, and they serve as useful lessons to apply to the competitive challenges of consumer-driven healthcare.

Retail Healthcare Takes Off

In 2012, more than *10 million patients* visited convenient-care clinics at the major retailers, a massive increase from just a few years prior. Walmart recently announced its ambition to become the largest provider of primary care in the United States. Figure 10.1 illustrates the growth in retail clinic use between 2007 and 2012.

Figure 10.1| The rise of retail clinic visits

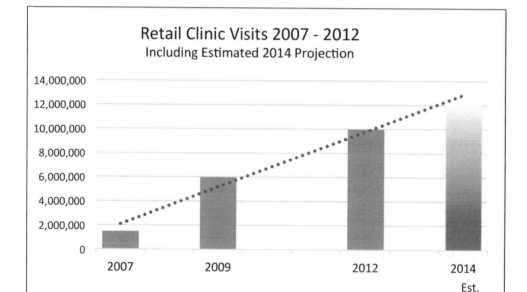

The successful encroachment of retail giants into the provider space plainly tells us that Americans want medical care in a convenient setting. They want it at a reasonable and transparent cost, and they want the care delivered in a timely fashion. That's it. It's not all that complex and not at all surprising.

Marc Baer, Target's senior director of managed care, recently remarked, "In a time when health plans and benefit providers are trying to figure out how to get people to engage in staying healthy or getting healthy, we fundamentally believe that simplicity, plus a great guest experience, will lead to engagement." That's a good lesson for those in the provider sector to learn.

Service Line Approach to Combat New Competitors

Let's face it: Up until the late eighties, the provider side of healthcare was fairly stagnant in terms of new competition. Then, in the early nineties, corresponding with the successful operation of Wall Street-backed healthcare enterprises, the competitive landscape shifted and niche players made a strong case for carving up the profitable segments of the business.

As a result, over the past 15 to 20 years, hospitals and health systems have become preoccupied with competitive threats from specialty hospitals, physician ventures, convenient care clinics, and a wide array of single-service providers (what Regina Herzog called "focused factories"). These agents of change pose a serious threat to legacy providers, to the point that progressive providers have embraced the approach and either partnered with specialty enterprises or developed specialty services within their own portfolios.

These partnerships have proven to be beneficial in many cases, but teaming up with retail-oriented enterprises doesn't mean that legacy providers have mastered the art of the consumer. Understanding consumer interest, motivation, and needs requires a wholesale shift in thought and operations and application of a well-defined market-driven strategy.

The lesson for legacy providers is this: Don't focus on the venue; focus on the benefits the consumer derives from the venue. Focus on the model offered. Healthcare executives caught up in the art of the deal don't recognize the shifting of market dynamics and often miss the opportunity to connect with the consumer.

The market advantage of retail-savvy competitors

What advantages do these relatively new retail healthcare providers bring to the mix? The list is short, but it represents a clear and immediate danger to healthcare providers who have not yet embraced a consumer model:

- They are singularly focused on one specialty or service line (SL)

- They often have financial support and operational input from physicians

- They are easily identified and positioned in the minds of patients

- They are often aggressive and savvy about marketing

- They often don't have the same degree of social responsibility (e.g., charity care and mission-driven objectives) as do hospitals and health systems

- They can easily maneuver in a changing market

- They usually operate much more efficiently

Large hospitals and health systems have long believed that their strength lay in their depth and breadth, providing an inherently superior model. However, the data presented in Figure 10.1 clearly shows that consumers/patients are asking the question: "Who cares about the girth of an organization? I'm interested in the extent to which you are meeting my needs."

The market advantage that health systems once assumed would always accrue to their benefit has eroded, thanks to the success of these consumer-focused, retail-savvy and sometimes behemoth (as in the case of the big-box stores) competitors. As insurance exchanges take shape and consumers are more empowered and active, market-savvy competitors will likely pose an even greater threat.

This is not only on account of the access, convenience, and timeliness factors: There is also the consumer-friendly element of heightened pricing transparency. Market-facing competitors have long provided upfront (usually considerably lower) costs and, as a result, patients perceive higher value for the price of the service.

In a consumer-driven environment, pricing is (practically) everything

Many legacy providers still don't price their services in a logical and understandable fashion. They raise the issue of "chargemaster calculus," citing that it's too complex to provide individualized pricing for selective services.

You read it here: The chargemaster—as we know it—will become extinct within five to eight years for the majority of services available from large-scale competitors. That doesn't mean providers will have stopped using it as an excuse for greater transparency and retail pricing. It just means that those providers will be left behind in the competitive environment.

Many of these competitors are focused on a single specialty or SL (i.e., cardiovascular center or an orthopedic hospital). The SL structure—with its emphasis on treating each designated category as its own individual enterprise— is the optimal model and architecture for competing with the niche players and entrepreneurial ventures.

SL Structure Helps Thwart Competition

As noted, an SL structure actually provides one of the best operating and organizational structures to anticipate specialized competition. If an SL structure is in place and dedicated managers are assigned to the core SLs, it's a pretty good bet that the SL manager and his or her SL team will be among the first to know about any potential competitive threats.

Part of that SL manager's job is to keep track of and communicate market dynamics to key stakeholders. This needs to be done throughout the organization, upward to senior management (sometimes rising to the board level), across to colleagues involved in the SL structure, and down to associates on the front lines who provide services within the SL framework. To do that, the SL manager will be in constant contact with the key stakeholders pertaining to the SL. This includes physicians, both those loyal to the facility and those more aligned with the competition.

Southwest case study

Some years ago, a rapidly growing and attractive market in the Southwest was home to two large health systems. One was an entrenched religious system that had a solid reputation and the leading market position. The other was an investor-owned system that had been formed during the high-merger era of the late 1990s and was gradually gaining share on the nonprofit system. Both systems had strong cardiac programs that accounted for a disproportionate share of revenue and margin.

Given the dynamics of the market—two strong systems, heavy managed care, younger-than-average population, and more than one strong cardiology group—the setting did not look all that favorable for a cardiac hospital to thrive. This market would not seem to be too fertile for the likes of a specialty hospital. Yet, one of the cardiology hospital firms (headquartered in the Southeast) opened a facility in the market, and within two years, the facility had assumed the number one position in terms of consumer awareness. In addition, the heart hospital had taken about one-third of the volume away from the larger, more entrenched systems in the area. In doing so, the smaller, SL-specific hospital provided some valuable lessons for all facing similar market dynamics.

In essence, the specialized facility was able to come into an established market and create a perception among the public that it was the top-of-mind place to seek care for anything related to the heart. This was true for diagnoses ranging from diagnostic testing to heart surgery. Why? Because the singular medical focus (or at least main focus) was the heart. By capturing the public's attention and awareness, the specialty hospital also was in a better position to negotiate with managed care companies and work with employers on services ranging from executive physicals to cardiac rehabilitation. There were many lessons to be learned from this particular case study:

- Take all competition seriously, especially entities that threaten the core business and key SLs.

- Never underestimate a new market entrant due to size or experience.

- Never presume what the market wants or how the consumer will respond.

- Strike preemptively, not reactively. The enterprise that is first in terms of what marketers call "mindshare" will usually not be dislodged from that position. In this case, the specialty hospital—even though the last entrant into the market for this SL—was able to vault to first place in the consumer's mind due to its strategic positioning.

- Structure the competitive response and market position to match that of the competition, or—even better—to one-up the competition.

An interesting epilogue to this story is that the firm that launched this facility—and many like it across the country—eventually sold virtually all of its facilities. This particular entity was sold to the for-profit enterprise, which incorporated the specialty hospital into its portfolio and subsequently captured the lion's share of cardiology business in the area.

One prominent reason legacy hospitals and health systems have taken such a full-impact hit from competitors such as specialty players is that far too often they haven't had dedicated individuals or teams assigned to monitor the market. Consequently, in many instances, by the time senior executives in the legacy organization get word of a physician uprising, a competitive inroad, or a major defection, it's too late—a fait accompli for the encroaching competitor and, more often than not, a serious blow to the legacy provider's position in the market. As such, attempts to salvage the situation are too often stop-gap or reactive and therefore ineffective.

Look at what has happened in many of the markets where specialized competitors have entered. The responses have been anything but calculated and the subsequent success far from stellar. One faith-based hospital in Central California experienced a serious decline in its overall outpatient volume (including OP surgery) and ancillary service revenue as a result of several enterprising ventures backed by or comanaged with physicians in the area, and in particular one expanding outpatient surgery center. This hospital experienced a decline of more than 40% in outpatient-related services over the course of three years, due to the encroachment of the physician-backed enterprises. Obviously, this wave of competing ventures (virtually all of which were physician-owned) had a significant negative impact on the organization's bottom line and its overall financial position within its system.

The imperative of consumer/market research

As related to more recent competitors—the retail giants—how many times have the legacy institutions conducted market research in their market to calculate and project the economic impact on their organization? I have heard of precious few. More often than not, hospitals and health system executives pursue one of two strategies:

1. They attempt to replicate the model with a proprietary (home-grown) clinic or two of their own

2. They decide to partner with the retail giant

The former strategy has been only moderately successful for most of the organizations that have attempted it. The latter strategy has worked far better in a number of markets, but even then, it has not been sure-fire. In both models, I can count on my hand the number of times that the legacy organization conducted consumer research to test the viability and sustainability of either model.

Rather than trust the instincts of the executives or follow the prescribed operating models already in place, here's a novel idea: **ask your prospective patients**. It's not rocket science to consider and execute consumer research, but neither is it common practice in our industry. The lack of consumer market research is one of the most troubling, baffling, and glaring deficiencies in our approach to understand our key stakeholder group, the healthcare consumer. Fortunately, some of that is changing as progressive leaders of forward-thinking systems and hospitals recognize the need for taking the pulse of the individuals who will be purchasing and using their services.

An outstanding case in point involves one of the largest nonprofit systems in the nation headquartered in California. Prior to a major rebranding initiative in 2013, this system undertook extensive consumer research, with a considerable number of focus group sessions (creatively and effectively administered in a home setting) and more than 1,600 quantitative surveys (phone or email). The result was an elegant and effective brand rollout that resonated with consumers (surprise), achieved the system's goals for communicating its organizational position, and strengthened its overall brand. So, here's what needs to happen in regard to effective consumer/market research:

- Identify the key audiences that will derive benefit from the new products or services.

- Decide what you want to derive from the research, whether it's validation of the value of the new services/products, information regarding elements of the program (location, pricing, hours, etc.), or key messages regarding the new offerings. Then ensure that the research will answer those core questions and produce actionable findings.

- Hire a professional market research firm to assist in developing the survey tools, both quantitative (email or phone surveys) and qualitative (focus groups).

- Involve senior leadership in the research, especially in the focus groups. These can be quite telling and revealing.

- Summarize the key findings of the market research, and demonstrate how those findings helped shape the eventual structure of the new services/products and positioning to the key stakeholders (i.e., consumers, physicians, and community).

This particular example involves research conducted at the broader organizational level—in this case the system—but market research is just as relevant and as beneficial at the SL level.

Market Reconnaissance on a Focused Basis, and the Need for Preemptive Strategy

The best time to develop strategy is early in the process, when several variables still are in play and multiple options are available. When strategy is planned at the 11th hour, however, with very few options available, the execution is usually short-sighted, overly expensive, and predictably reactive. It is just the nature of the planning process. One of the greatest benefits of an SL strategy is that if it is well organized, high profile, and ultimately accountable, it buys you time not only for planning counterstrategy, but also for preempting competitive threats in the first place.

Many healthcare leaders have yet to recognize the notion that highly effective, dedicated SL managers will earn their salaries several times over just focusing on market dynamics and competitive activity. If the SL manager has too many other responsibilities—even in terms of line management responsibility—the odds of that manager being tapped into the competitive market are slim. He or she is more likely to concentrate efforts on internal management than market focus, and although the former is highly important, the latter cannot be ignored or dismissed. That noted, if the organization selects SL managers who can effectively manage internal dynamics and monitor the competitive landscape, a relatively high salary for a middle manager is well worth the investment.

Take a look at the math: Within a year or two of executing on his or her business plan, an SL manager earning in the $80,000 to $160,000 salary range should realistically expect to realize incremental net revenue in the $2 to $4 million range for the SL, with contribution margins of $800,000 to $1.6 million, and net operating income (bottom line performance) of several hundred thousand dollars. That applies to competition that currently exists as well as to competitors that may be in the offing.

Unfortunately, too many senior executives believe that this kind of market reconnaissance is the purview and prerogative of marketing directors or department managers, who have other responsibilities as well. Granted, some organizations do have individuals who consider it part of their responsibility to keep their finger on the pulse—and some of them achieve admirable success in so doing. However, there is often the dilution and distraction factor for most individuals whose role is either so widespread (i.e., marketing director) or so operationally in-depth (i.e., department director).

Whatever the reason or the distraction, the traditional hospital organizational structure is not well-suited for anticipating competitive threats or for successfully countering such threats once they become a reality in the market. If you don't believe that statement, think about your own organization, and how effectively your hospital or system has responded to specialty players, physician-backed enterprises, or convenient care clinics. If the honest answer is "quite effectively," count yourself in a very elite minority.

And not to sound this note too many times, but with heightened consumerism on the imminent horizon, the need for such accurate and anticipatory market reconnaissance will be all the more important—there will be less room for error and higher stakes for everyone involved.

SL Managers and the Role of Market Intelligence

An organization with a functioning SL model can and should position itself to take advantage of its structure for gathering competitive reconnaissance. SL managers should provide regular reports on competitor initiatives, marketing tactics/campaigns, and new products or services offered by the competitors. This can be done either formally through business plan updates or informally through some type of periodic review. A rigorous and systematic process or system for reporting such competitive activity gives senior management a more accurate picture of what is occurring in their market, as well as what they might anticipate. It also gives senior executives invaluable guidance for their strategic planning and capital allocation decisions.

Without ongoing and robust market intelligence, the outcome too often is rapid-fire development and implementation of a reactive strategy (which is really not that strategic by definition), or a suboptimal execution, because the counter-response is executed in haste—without proper lead time, market research, and stakeholder input.

The truth is that many of the pitfalls of faulty initiatives and flawed strategy would be avoided if the process and structure existed for periodic reports from the field. Yet few organizations actually institute a competitive assessment process. Many organizations do not even have a formalized strategic planning process, including some of the larger and more financially viable for-profit organizations, although that has changed somewhat in recent years.

Nonetheless, this begs the question: "Well, if some of the large for-profit companies and their hospitals do not have structured and rigorous planning as part of their regimen, why should any organizations bother?" One empirically based answer can be found in the roller-coaster history of both investor-owned and some large-scale, nonprofit hospitals and health systems. Look at most of the well-known firms—particularly the for-profit enterprises—and you will observe a trend of peak-and-valley financial performance. Granted, some of this is to be expected, given the nature of the industry and the unpredictability of many of the variables that affect healthcare. Yet, the counterargument is that a more volatile industry should actually lend itself to even greater time and effort when it comes to strategic planning.

Given the imminent changes expected related to increasing consumer empowerment and the heightened impact of market forces and government regulation, effective market reconnaissance and competitive intelligence will become even more important. That element of business strategy and effective market positioning is really best facilitated and orchestrated at the SL level.

How to Gather Intelligence on Competitors

A good SL manager will become as familiar with the competition as the employees who work there. In the consumer-goods industry, product or brand managers spend a great deal of time studying the moves and motives of their key competitors. They keep tabs on what the competitors are doing from both an operational and marketing standpoint, so they can not only anticipate the impact on the market but they can be prepared to respond in a way that will effectively neutralize the competition's efforts.

In healthcare, of course, this often takes on the look or feel of me-too initiatives. Let's be honest: We have earned a reputation for being an industry of lemmings that follow the competitor located across the street or the seemingly successful hospital across the state. This type of reaction often is just that—a reaction—that is not grounded in thoughtful/methodical business practice or carefully planned execution.

The value of an SL orientation when it comes to competing—especially against smaller and more nimble players—is that it subdivides the organization into strategic business units (SBU) that can more effectively compete because the manager overseeing those SLs is given the authority and the accountability to track competitor movement and then to respond (not react) accordingly. Of course, the SL managers keep senior management well informed on both competitor movement and the recommended strategy to counter and contend with the competition. This is an integral part of their job function, not something that is left to chance or eleventh-hour reaction.

In essence, an SL structure gives managers a more acute awareness that they are responsible not only for their own SL but for the competitor's business as well. They fully understand that what the competition does will have a direct impact on their business. This concept of "managing the competition" is not a notion that is prevalent in the hospital field, but it is in other industries. As our sector becomes more market-driven, I believe this attitude and approach will gain more traction and will pay valuable dividends for those organizations that understand and practice it.

Not all competitors should be treated as combatants, nor should they necessarily be regarded as such (this is, after all, a field noted for more civility than most industries, due to faith-based institutions and nonprofit origins). Along those lines, then, one outcome of monitoring actions by competitors may be to offer a strategy involving collaboration. The concept of "coopetition"—cooperating or collaborating while still competing—has taken greater hold in our industry over the past two decades. Some of this is driven by the realization that there are market synergies to be realized from effective collaboration, and some of it is due to the changing landscape, especially under the umbrella of population health management.

As it plays out, this type of collaboration and linking up—either financially, virtually, or some combination of both—is likely to increase once insurance exchanges are actualized. That was the experience in Massachusetts when the Massachusetts Connector (that state's version of the exchange) was implemented. Jon Kingsdale, who oversaw that program, observed that "the rapid consolidation of providers with providers, payers with providers, and payers with payers" was one of the market dynamics "that surprised him most."

Given the experience in Massachusetts, we are likely to see the same market dynamic across the country over the next few years.

Creative Positioning Tactics

Joint ventures with physicians

An example of this comes into play with possible joint venture between members of the medical staff. As physicians experience declining practice incomes and greater demands on their time, they are seeking to gain more control over their lives and their economic future. Consequently, many are splintering off and developing enterprises that directly compete with the hospitals or health systems that have provided them a venue to practice their profession for decades.

Although some healthcare executives view this as a kind of treason, or at the least a competitive threat, savvy executives will anticipate the interests and needs of key members of their medical staff and begin evaluating opportunities for partnership with the doctors on ventures that are mutually beneficial and legally permissible. These kinds of ventures offer all parties the option to collaborate rather than compete outright, and whereas the ultimate outcome may not be as economically attractive for the hospital or health system, it may prove to be better than losing the large share of business that would migrate away from the hospital to the physician's office. Such an arrangement may even produce synergistic opportunities for both parties.

Furthermore, the hospital or health system that incorporates the notion of faithfully monitoring and managing the competition will find that its overall strategy improves. This should occur as the organization undertakes a more structured and calculated approach to assessing and analyzing the strategy of its competition. Again, in many industries, competitor analysis is fundamental. In healthcare, it is too often limited to the annual (or even less frequent) review of the market as part of the environmental assessment. However, if such assessment and analysis occurs only on an infrequent and limited basis, the significant moves of competitors—either existing or possible—will not be detected in a timely fashion.

Case Study of a Joint Venture for Imaging Services

One major hospital system in the South determined that rather than risk the loss of more volume migrating to imaging centers, it would partner with the largest radiology group in the area. Although some executives feel that to give up a section of the market, or a sizable piece of the pie, is untenable, many are realizing that it is better to retain a segment of the high-margin imaging market (by partnering with physicians) than to risk losing the major percentage of the imaging business.

In the case of the system in the South, their gambit paid off. Not only were they able to retain a fairly significant segment of the market, the radiologists favored the initial arrangement so much that they invited the health system to participate in more such ventures. They valued the managerial expertise and marketing savvy that the large system brought to the joint enterprise. Consequently, the venture was a win-win-win, with eventual satisfaction and success for the physicians, the hospital system, and area patients, who received more convenient service at a lower cost and in a more expedited fashion.

Physician employment as positioning strategy

In these times when more physicians are seeking employment by the larger institution, the same fundamental dynamic applies. An SL manager/director who is in tune with the professional interests and business strategy of the physicians aligned with that particular SL will anticipate the group or individual physician's interest in employment. If astutely monitored and addressed, this will occur **before** the bidding war between competing hospitals begins.

In some cases, employment may be a presumed approach to meet the physician's interests, but in reality, other options (just as beneficial and perhaps less economically involved) may be developed to help the physician or physician group achieve its economic and business practice aims. Sadly, we've seen in recent years a kind of land rush mentality where physicians have "persuaded" hospital and health system executives to purchase their practices and provide an employment structure. Granted, some of these may be mutually beneficial, but a fair number are reminiscent of the deals that were constructed in the mid- to late nineties, during the infamous years of "integrated delivery systems."

As we now know in painful retrospect, most of those deals were financially unmerited and operationally unwise, and they have subsequently come unraveled. I rather suspect we'll see the same outcome with a fair number of these arrangements, particularly as we enter the cost-constrained world of accountable care and population management. However, to the credit of hospitals and health systems, some have learned their lesson, recognizing that their managerial practice and style do not overlay well on a physician practice. Consequently, they have carefully structured the arrangements around mutually beneficial incentives. In some cases they have also engaged the expertise of professional practice managers. In fact, one emerging subsegment in the provider sector is the outsourced management of purchased physician practices. My prediction is that this will be one of the most sought-after and successful offshoots of the entire employed-physician phenomenon.

The key point here, though, is that a savvy SL manager or director can help avoid some of that economic pain by anticipating the general interests of the physicians and clinicians within the purview of his/her SL.

As with so many components of SL structure, the SL manager and his or her colleagues bring great value to the organization in terms of the information they provide and all the discipline they exhibit. If the SL structure is adequately and accurately functioning, the competitive response—ranging from aggressive competition to possible collaboration—will be more readily identified and more easily achieved.

Conclusion

The notion of competition in the American healthcare system is as entrenched as it is productive. An effective and robust SL architecture offers an excellent framework for assessing an organization's competitive position and then determining the optimal strategy. In an era of market-savvy and highly powerful competitors who understand the consumer much better than hospital or health system executives can reasonably hope to, an SL strategy can help transform a larger, inflexible, and slow-moving legacy organization into a market-responsive and consumer-focused entity that can compete more effectively.

Additionally, a dedicated SL manager, supported by a multidisciplinary team, can more readily anticipate market needs and more successfully anticipate and respond to competitive threats. Some options available include collaboration or even "coopetition," where the hospital or health system chooses to partner with a specialty player, enterprising physician group, or retail giant in the convenient care clinic space. Whatever the selected mechanism or model for competitive response, an SL structure is an excellent organizational framework for matching the resources of the organization to the demands of the market.

11

The Inherent Value of Disciplined Business Planning

Once the structure and framework have been established and the individuals are selected to fulfill the roles, the next step is to create a sophisticated and detailed business plan. Developing a rigorous business plan for each service line (SL) and revising it annually are essential to your success. Unfortunately, the individual SL business plans are sometimes overlooked, and periodic reviews are neglected.

The organizational value of crafting a business plan for each strategic business unit cannot be overstated. SL-specific plans allow the organization to break down the system wide strategic plan into actionable, detailed "tactical" plans. Far too many hospitals and health systems suffer a disconnect between the all-encompassing strategic plan and its eventual execution because they haven't established a mechanism to "operationalize" the plan at the market-facing, SL level.

The SL Business Plan

Disciplined business planning at the SL level pays meaningful dividends across the enterprise, by documenting and recognizing achieved goals and successfully implemented initiatives. Let's take a look at the characteristics of an effective SL business plan:

1. It is an **action-oriented document** that flows out of the enterprise wide strategic plan. The strategic plan and the SL business plans should exhibit an interdependency that makes both documents more robust.

2. The SL business plan cycle should **sync with the strategic plan cycle**. At the outset, the strategic plan for the organization will precede the SL plans, serving as the root document for the SL plans.

3. Additionally, the SL plans should **support the overall strategic direction** and goals of the organization. The day may come when the organization must decide which areas have greater strategic relevance and therefore which SLs will receive the appropriate resources.

As counterintuitive as it may seem, SL plan diversions from the strategic plan are not all that uncommon. But failing to align the two could mean that even considerable success within the SL does not advance the overall goals of the organization. In other words, SL business plans may occasionally be at odds with the organizational strategic plan. Obviously, that's not a good situation.

When diverging plans create a less-than-ideal situation, the outcome can be described as a *subsegment overshadowing the full complement*. In the retail world, this situation might play out in a shopping mall where one high-profile store stands out and performs well at the expense of the entire mall. In the long run, it matters little that the one store is a star. The mall may eventually shutter its operations for failure to meet its broader goals.

More than a few hospitals and health systems have enjoyed stellar individual programs or SLs but struggled on the whole as a result of SL goals that were incompatible with organizational strategic objectives. You can avoid this outcome by ensuring that your SL business plans are consistent with the overarching goals and objectives of the larger organization.

Integrating SL Plans into the Strategic Plan

The task then for senior executives is to create a broad-based strategic plan for the hospital or health system that provides delineated market-course direction and operational parameters. These guiding parameters should include:

- Financial targets
- Volume goals
- Capital availability
- Staffing resources
- Market share expectations

If integrated effectively, the SL business plans can both contribute to and benefit from the umbrella strategy outlined in the organization's strategic plan.

You may ask why any hospital or health system would neglect to synchronize the two levels of the planning process. This failure occurs for a variety of reasons:

- In some instances, the organization has not developed a long-range strategic plan, which obviously makes the connection with individual SL plans problematic, if not impossible.

- The organization's "strategic" plan is not all that strategic or robust in the first place. Rather than clearly outlining the performance glide path for the organization and specific activities and time frames required to achieve that trajectory, the plan is rife with sweeping mission statements and objectives presented as platitudes. It lacks realistic, time-boxed imperatives and measurable objectives.

- Senior leaders in the organization fail to communicate the need to effectively link the plans. In too many cases, this is not the result of an oversight or lack of clarity, but a cultural desire to keep the strategic plan cloistered within tight ranks and not cascaded throughout the organization as it should be. The concept of "need to know" with limited access to critical strategic direction and information is a recipe for failed communications and is usually both unsound and unjustified.

In the case of an organization that does not have a strategic plan, or has one that doesn't offer clear guidance for the individual plans, it's possible to proceed without the benefit of an overarching, direction-providing document. Organizations faced with the need to develop a few key strategic business units, such as cardiology, may launch with a business plan for just the individual SL, but it will provide fewer parameters against which to gauge the SL's link to the overall strategic direction of the enterprise.

For example, when the SL team suggests (through its detailed business plan) that what the SL really needs is a new center of excellence to provide differentiation from the competition, an organization that does not have a substantive strategic plan has no framework in which to evaluate such a recommendation in the broader context. In this case, the center of excellence in cardiology may sound reasonable and even alluring, but if the organization has no broader context in which to evaluate that recommended strategy, it may draw critical resources and capital allocation away from higher-priority initiatives, such as developing a clinical integration strategy.

In essence, a strategic plan offers direction and provides critical "guard rails" or parameters for the individual services within the hospital or health system. Without it, competition for scarce capital and other resources is similar to the Old West version of the land rush: the first, loudest, or most aggressive manager to lay a claim is awarded the resources and declared the winner.

The new world order under an accountable care model, with the need for effective population health, and against the backdrop of rising consumerism will require even greater attention to and coordination/synchronization with the organization's long-range plan to realize lasting success in this new market environment.

Basic Elements of the Strategic Plan

Ideally, your organization's strategic plan will be completed and in place prior to the completion—or at least adoption—of the SL business plans. This vital precursor will save a great deal of disruption and inefficient resource allocation down the road.

One of the biggest mistakes that executives and planners make in crafting their strategic plans is to gather mountains of marginally useful data that may be interesting but not all that relevant to the final goals, strategies, and measures of success. Unfortunately, this is where some executive teams get bogged down. It's a modern twist on the poet Samuel Taylor Coleridge's famous line, "Water, water everywhere, and not a drop to drink." As it relates to modern-day strategic planning, far too often we face a strategic plan with "Data, data everywhere, and not a *thought to think.*"

Remember this: The strategic plan does not need to be worthy of eventual placement in the healthcare hall of fame. Good strategic plans are readable and digestible documents, rather than Tolkien-length tomes.

At its essence, a workable strategic plan (and, to a large extent, an SL business plan) should include the following elements:

- Environmental analysis or overview (relevant conditions in the local market)
- Market assumptions (for major players, competitors, potential partners, stakeholder groups such as major employers, insurance companies, and others)
- Critical success factors (those four or five imperatives that absolutely have to happen to achieve success)
- Goals for the organization (over a three- to five-year time frame, or whatever the plan calls for)
- Strategies to achieve the goals
- Assignments and measures to gauge success (accountability matrix)

- Action plans with detailed time allocations for each one

Your plans can include much more than the above components, but this list is a good starting point. Now let's look at creating a business plan for your SL.

Basic Elements of an SL Business Plan

The difference between an SL business plan and the strategic plan is the SL plan's singular focus on one subsegment of the organization's portfolio and its corresponding emphasis on tactical execution. The SL plan can and should be much more "on the tarmac" so to speak, whereas the strategic plan tends to hover at 30,000 feet. Consequently, the SL business plan can get into significantly more detail than a strategic plan and should involve a more thorough analysis of the operational components of the individual SL.

There are several elements to a typical SL plan, including environmental analysis, market assumptions, critical success factors, SL goals, strategies, and accountability.

Environmental analysis

This facet of the plan should focus on measuring the SL vis-a-vis its competition (existing as well as expected). It is absolutely imperative to gauge how the SL is positioned within the local or regional market. Consequently, this element of your business plan should involve a fairly exhaustive competitive analysis that would include both qualitative (perception) as well as quantitative (actual data) measures, which may call for very different strategies.

Note that perceived quality can be as important as actual—at least in the short run. There was a time when actual quality was not as relevant, but with the push for publicizing quality data, hospitals need to be acutely aware of how they stack up in comparison with the competition. The rise of the retail model, with more financially and intellectually engaged consumers, will make comparable quality data more relevant as well.

For example, one hospital in a large metropolitan area had very good indexes for mortality and morbidity relative to the competition in the area. However, due to years of positioning as the "safety net" hospital in the area, its perceived quality was significantly below that of the other facilities as measured by consumer research. This hospital's problem, then, is one of communication, not of clinical improvement. For this particular facility, its strategy needs to center around education or promotion, rather than merely operational improvement. Many hospitals—especially inner city hospitals—face this very challenge.

The value of having at least two measures—actual quality and perceived quality—for many stakeholder groups should be patently evident. And this is not just relevant for consumers or patients. The same analysis could be plotted for physicians, employers, community leaders, and even health plans. This dual analysis offers a sense of position—both perceptual as well as actual—and can be used to craft a strategy to address relative market position in each area.

A caution about environmental analysis

Although it is important to provide the backdrop against which (and within which) the organizations must operate, many organizations spend too much energy on the environmental analysis. The environmental assessment doesn't need to be all that extensive to formulate reasonable goals and sound strategies. The bulk of the time should be invested in understanding the essential things that must be achieved (critical success factors) and then crafting goals and strategies that reflect that determination.

The environmental analysis metrics should closely follow other the metrics identified earlier in the book, as the success of the SL will be gauged and the objectives will be established based on them.

> **Note** The most elaborate and sophisticated environmental analysis means nothing if the organization fails to grasp its core imperatives, understand its key audiences, and execute its essential strategies.

Market assumptions

In this section of the business plan, the management team identifies the market factors that are likely to have significant bearing on the SL and what to expect from them going forward. In other words, given the best information available to the SL team and others within the organization, what is the expected trajectory for these entities or players in the market over the next few years?

This list doesn't need to be an exhaustive or overly detailed projection; avoid investing an inordinate amount of time in research and consensus building. The list should simply serve the purpose of providing a sense of what is expected from these key players. Enterprises or entities to consider in this analysis should include:

- Hospitals in the area that provide similar services to the line in question.

- Niche players such as specialty hospitals, ambulatory surgery centers, or entrepreneurial ventures that currently are or might soon get into the specific line of business. (A case in point would be convenience care clinics or imaging services in retail settings.)

- Physicians or physician groups with a direct impact or influence on the SL.

- Managed care plans or payers that exercise financial influence.

- Government regulation or reimbursement that relates directly to the SL.

- Technological considerations and innovations integral to the SL in question.

- Other activities or ventures that might be associative or collaborative, such as complementary services that might exert influence on this line (i.e., hospice services for oncology).

- Local political initiatives or civic actions that might have some effect, such as a move to form coalitions for specific disease categories or initiatives focused on wellness or healthy living.

Critical success factors

Critical success factors are those operational components that an organization must complete in order to achieve its objectives. These are the absolutes within the plan, the essentials.

One example that applies to nearly every hospital and health system is **staffing imperatives**. In this category, a hospital might select benchmarks (e.g., peer hospital, or statewide average) for staffing ratios, vacancy rates, turnover rates, and so forth, and note its position relative to the determined benchmarks.

For many hospitals and health systems, a certain level of **profitability or financial stability** would be listed as a critical success factor, as that is how organizations are evaluated by governing bodies that oversee local management. In this regard, then, a critical success factor might be maintaining a certain level of profitability or an established margin threshold.

Along the same lines, **cost control** or **operational efficiency** also might be delineated for a hospital in these times of limited (and diminishing) resources.

Faced with market volume growth—caused by an aging or rising population in the area—many organizations often list **sources of capital** as a critical success factor. To this end, the critical success considerations may involve forthright assessments of the organization's need to maintain a certain rating in the bond market.

For some facilities, **physical plant capacity** will be a critical success factor, given the aging of the population in the market and the increasing demand for inpatient or outpatient capacity.

Considering the emerging need for expanded physical capacity, many executives are facing the daunting issue of **capital constraints**, which is looming as one of the major dilemmas in the industry (and one of the driving forces behind the consolidation movement). In many markets, and within many boardrooms, reliable access to capital is becoming one of the biggest challenges facing senior leadership over the next five to 10 years.

The list of critical success factors to include in your plan should be no longer than five or six items. Here's an example from one hospital in the Upper Midwest:

1. Recruitment and retention of qualified personnel for the SL

2. Capital availability for SL projects

3. Quality of care—perceived and actual in this SL

4. Physician alignment relative to this line

5. Physical plant condition and competitiveness

6. Financial stability as measured by the SL profit and loss

Narrowing the list down to a manageable number of factors (preferably no more than seven) will require some effort to distill the crucial considerations down to the priorities. This is a valuable exercise in and of itself, somewhat like prioritizing the SLs. However, the inherent value in first assessing the vital considerations and then selecting those that are critical to success is that it sharpens the focus of the SL team. For at the end of the day, if those critical success factors are not realized, no matter what else the organization may do—as lofty and noble as it may be—it will not achieve its fundamental objectives and fulfill its core reason for existence.

SL goals

Next, list the goals or objectives for the coming year and then the next three to five years (to sync with the strategic plan). These goals should broadly align with the organization's plan and then be definitive and qualitative enough that they are measurable.

Too many organizations make goals that sound more like platitudes than performance targets. For example, a goal like "Continue to improve quality within the cardiology department" sounds very laudable and admirable, but it is difficult to define and difficult to measure, unless specific targets are established. For example, in this area, the business plan could call for the SL to achieve quality rankings in the top decile for that area.

It is far better to narrow a goal if that means being more specific in listing the target. For example, another goal might be to improve access to cardiovascular services in the community by bringing three new cardiologists and one new surgeon to the area within five years. The goal is easy to measure, easy to account for, and, assuming the shortage of physicians is a real need, easy to justify. Furthermore, such a goal will likely resonate with a number of stakeholder groups.

Examples of other goals that are somewhat broader in scope but still quantifiable include the following:

- Improve financial performance by increasing operation margin in this SL from 5% to 8% in two years

- Increase market share for the SL in question from 35% to 40% in four years

- Increase inpatient capacity for the SL by 20% in the next five years

- Improve favorable market perception by consumers by 10% as measured in market research surveys

- Improve favorable market perception among physicians by 10% as measured by the medical staff survey

- Improve favorable market perception among employers by 15% as measured in employer roundtable discussions/surveys

The goals can be more narrowly focused to factor in major developments within a particular SL, if deemed significant (enough) to the entire organization. For example, two SL–oriented goals that have broad implications would be incorporating a neuroscience SL into the organizational mix or completing construction of a new cancer center.

In these latter instances, the goals are broad enough that they will affect the entire system in terms of both capital allocation and managerial attention. Goals must have enough significance to capture the organization's imagination and enough definition to ensure that their accomplishment can be measured.

Strategies to achieve the goals

The strategies section should spell out the accompanying initiatives that will help the organization achieve its overarching goals. Some might argue that developing the neuroscience SL and the new cancer center actually are strategies (rather than goals), and perhaps this is true from a purist point of view. However, the goals of the organization should be derived as much for the motivation and momentum they produce as to satisfy an academic definition of an objective.

Consequently, I would argue that putting down the addition of a neuroscience SL as a goal (and something that is certain to consume a great deal of management time and attention) may be of greater value than a broader but less definitive goal. The ultimate decision on this is up to each management team.

The important thing to remember is that strategies are the broad actions necessary to accomplish or achieve the objectives—both for the organization overall and for the specific SL. For example, the goal of achieving market share growth will likely be achieved via a number of SL extensions, SL expansions, or supporting strategies. Perhaps the oncology line needs to expand into radiation therapy to increase its share, as well as improve its financial position. Another situation might involve a decision by the surgery SL to begin offering bariatric surgery to expand the line. These strategies can be included to achieve the overarching organizational objectives.

As with the goals, strategies should be given specific time frames for completion—and in the more detailed documents (which do not need to be shown to the board or governance bodies), which support the SL business plans and provide much more granular information, the specific details of the action plans should be defined clearly. The strategy section needs not be overly detailed but rather should be a document that is presented to senior management and board leadership and is understood as the type of information that deserves a great deal of attention, discussion, and frequent review.

The leaders of the organization need to present this information with the clear understanding and realization that the strategies outlined will result in the accomplishment of the broad goals of the organization.

Accountability

Although this section of the plan may not be as compelling or intellectually stimulating as the broad goals and bold strategies, this probably is the most difficult section, as it is the most demanding and often the most difficult to bring to fruition. This section is where the organization gets very granular. It may be relatively easy to spout off lofty goals, brilliant strategies, and crucial market factors, but fruition is in the details. This section will never be seen by the board (at least, I wouldn't recommend it), but it should be reviewed and monitored often by senior management.

The hard gravel road section should include timelines that spell out the stages of execution and achievement, as well as defining who is accountable. The detailed sections of the plan might also include guidepost measures that would help management assess whether the goals are being achieved and whether the strategies are proving successful. This facet of the plan often is overlooked or underreported, but that does not make periodic assessment any less essential. In fact, some organizations are moving toward project management to ensure that the implementation of the action plans is accomplished.

All this sounds like a somewhat daunting task, but business plans can be the basis of a disciplined approach to keeping the organization on track and helping ensure that management is fulfilling its stewardship to the community and to its stakeholders.

Conclusion

Many hospitals and health systems throughout the country engage in strategic planning, but too few organizations take the process of planning down to the SL level. However, the SL level is the point at which planning is actualized and, therefore, is the market-facing level at which it needs to occur. Due to the proximity of the consumer/patient to the services offered, this is also the level at which planning is likely to bear the greatest fruit, as this type of approach can most closely match the dynamics of the market and provide the sought-after competitive advantage.

There should be an element of symbiosis between the organization's strategic plan and its more detailed SL business plans. Whereas the strategic plan should drive the overarching direction of the hospital and health system, the SL business plans should support and sustain the broader goals and strategies of the strategic plans.

12

The Role of Marketing in Service Line Differentiation

The Role and Relevance of New Competitors

One of the greatest advantages of the service line (SL) structure relates to competitive positioning. As discussed in prior chapters, hospitals and health systems face increasing pressure from new entrants to the market, such as niche players (with physician ownership or involvement), big-box retail enterprises (Walmart or CVS) and Web-based entities (ZocDocs, iTriage, etc.). These new players bring a level of focus and flexibility that traditional competitors, such as the hospital across the street, or the health system within the metro area, rarely have exhibited.

Whether the competition is a nimble new player or a large legacy type, service line management (SLM) can help you compete more effectively and more decisively.

The Inestimable Value of Astute Marketing

The first wave of product line/SLM was misinterpreted as merely a marketing play. It is *not* a fundamental reason for the SL model—but it is an important aspect of it.

Too few executives in this field understand the true nature of marketing. I worked for a CEO who couldn't say "marketing" without grinding his teeth. Although his position and interpretation may have been more strident than most, he is not alone. These responses are due in part to the misapplication of marketing tools, tactics, and resources over the past three decades in the provider sector. It may also be attributable to the fact that the economic benefit of marketing initiatives (the return on investment, if you will) is not as easily documented and validated in healthcare as in other industries.

Still, the fact remains that marketing is integral to the successful implementation of the model. This is even truer in light of the emerging competition mentioned previously, and given the rise of the consumer. In essence, it is a new world that healthcare executives now must consider and confront, as they allocate decreasing resources in an increasingly challenged market environment.

In many—if not most—industries, the SL manager is drawn from the marketing function. In healthcare, however, the SL leader has tended to have either a clinical or a general administrative background. If this is the case in your organization, the SL manager or director should ensure that marketing plays a key role on the SL matrix team. This again illustrates the value of a matrix structure in which several functions and individuals contribute to the initial strategy and ongoing execution, which we took a close look at in Chapter 9.

Several elements of the marketing function are vital to successful SL implementation:

- **Market research**—Assessing and addressing the consumer's wants and needs is pivotal. It will be addressed in greater depth in this chapter.

- **Communication**—This core activity is vital for every SL and to each audience. However, marketing staff members often are the professionals within the organization charged with implementing the communication plan and message.

- **Competitive intelligence**—In most instances, the marketing staff is the group most aware of competitive maneuvers due to market reconnaissance, promotional initiatives, or advertising campaigns.

- **Promotion**—This element comes into play in various forms, from highlighting existing services to publicizing new programs.

- **Presentation (or packaging)**—Marketing experts should have a good sense for how best to position the services and products within the SL to the customers and other key audiences (e.g., physicians or family members).

- **Distribution**—Marketing experts should understand channels of distribution, which in healthcare may involve new delivery settings or revamping and revising existing facilities and enterprises.

- **Product development**—Again, marketing staff should be skilled at anticipating the needs of consumers when it comes to extending the SL with new services or expanding the customer base (i.e., tapping new market segments) for the various services offered within the SL.

The Need for Effective Market Research

One case in point is the application of market research, a highly integral and directional facet of the marketing which, as we've discussed, is not used as often in healthcare as in other industries. Yet well-conducted market research can be invaluable in assessing the inherent interest and probable outcome of new products or revamped services within the individual SL.

Organizations in every industry are able to avoid missteps and misfires when they take the time and spend the money to conduct market research prior to launching an initiative, or even promoting a particular service. Failure to do so can result in expensive miscalculations and embarrassing failures.

The cost of foregoing market research

One example comes to mind within this industry—namely, the push in the late nineties toward vertical integration with physicians. Across the nation, hospitals and health systems suffered sizable financial losses in their failed attempts to develop integrated delivery systems that were designed to provide more interface and interdependence with doctors.

Unfortunately, very little market research was conducted in terms of testing the concept in preemptive fashion with doctors and other key players in the field. As one physician, who no doubt spoke for many of his colleagues, said, "If [the administration] had asked me about the idea, I could have told them it would not work. But they never asked." The financial losses and resulting strained relations (between physicians and hospital executives) might have been avoided if just a little more basic research had been conducted. The truth is that, like a sequel to a B movie, we are seeing instances of this very dynamic playing out again with the rush to employ physicians in recent years. While this can be a viable and even essential strategy, the fact is that many of these deals (between hospital/ health system and physician group) are being completed with the same void of level-setting, preemptive research that we saw in the nineties. Conducting such research *prior* to consummating those relationships would no doubt improve the final agreements and ensure their long-term viability.

When it comes to launching a new service or considering a new fundamental direction for the SL, simply asking questions of those involved can produce valuable prelaunch insights and even essential epiphanies. Market research is especially relevant when it comes to dealing with a new model or application that involves a service or a delivery channel outside the norm.

Delivery channel disaster

In the late 1990s, a large for-profit hospital chain decided that it would offer maternity products in several malls throughout the country. However, marketing staff members never bothered to ask potential customers if they thought the concept was viable, or if they—the prospective customers—would value the venue and the basic idea of purchasing such products in a retail setting. The result was a major marketing meltdown. What was envisioned to grow to at least 20 retail settings in major metropolitan markets failed so colossally in the inaugural venture that the entire project was scrapped within weeks of the first store's opening in southern Florida.

In this instance, the executives in charge of execution presumed that the idea was sound and the concept would succeed (wrong!). As with so many similarly failed marketing forays and ill-executed ventures, a little pre-launch market research would have provided valuable insight into how the consumer would respond, and the healthcare organization could have avoided a significant expenditure and a major embarrassment. The consumers would have basically validated what some marketing-savvy experts would have intuited from the start: Why would people purchase a highly situation-dependent and setting-specific product from sales clerks not experienced clinicians, and in a general retail setting? In hindsight it seems so obvious, and yet as the adage goes, hindsight is usually 20-20. The value of market research is that it provides marketing and SL leaders the opportunity to engage the benefits of hindsight…through empirically tested consumer foresight. That, in essence, is what good marketing research does.

Diversification failures

Another example of that hypothesis could be found in the many failed attempts at diversification in the late eighties and early nineties within the industry. In those heady days, some hospitals mistakenly believed that diversification initiatives like laundry services, topflight restaurants, catering, and so forth would succeed. Unfortunately, many of these ventures did not fare well, and not only did they result in financial losses, they also were a diversion and distraction of managerial time and attention. Yet if the initial research had been conducted with key audiences (namely, prospective customers), many of the missteps could have been minimized, if not avoided altogether.

The ill-fated ventures of the past are worth revisiting now that many hospitals and health systems once again are looking to broaden revenue streams and diversify portfolios. It's not that the concept is a flawed one, or that the idea of moving into more retail settings is at all mistaken. Rather, testing the water with the proposed service or model and in the new setting is even more relevant today than it was 10 to 20 years ago. As noted earlier, highly successful systems—nonprofit and for-profit alike—have demonstrated the value of portfolio diversification, whether horizontal, vertical, or diagonal. Yet even to this day, many of these ventures lack the "testing the water" application of market research, which is too bad, as you'd think we would have learned our lesson.

Research as the voice of reason

To paraphrase one of Steve Jobs' most oft-cited managerial maxims: In his career, he was perhaps proudest of some of the things he chose *not* to do. We can see that wisdom play out by looking at a midsize hospital system in the Southwest that was considering a foray into the alternative medicine field.

The executives in this particular hospital system determined that because alternative medicine represented a very new operating model for their organization, they needed to survey the customer base to better understand the mind-set and the expectations of the purchaser. They conducted several focus group research sessions among heavy and moderate users of alternative medicine therapies such as message therapy, herbal treatments, and acupuncture.

These sessions, in which the executives viewed the proceedings behind one-way mirrors (as is typical for focus group sessions), proved to be highly illuminating. The findings produced by the focus groups ran counter to the delivery model the managers originally planned to implement. Focus group participants told the research facilitator they wanted and *expected* the alternative therapies to be offered in a setting that was starkly different from the traditional medical environment. They wanted wood floors, live plants, and soothing music playing in the background. They definitely did not want these therapies administered in a hospital-like or traditional physician-office setting.

Before the research, some of the hospital system leaders planned to expand their existing urgent care centers to offer the alternative modalities in those venues. The market research offered them an invaluable dose of reality. Consequently, they were able to avoid a major misstep in delivery setting and avert a financial disaster—just by spending a few thousand dollars to ask prospective patients what they expected and desired.

Decades ago, the legendary professor and marketing guru, Phillip Kotler, defined marketing as "The satisfaction of human needs and wants through the offering of products and services," or stated another way, "meeting the needs of the customer." To do that effectively, it's almost always a good idea to ask the customer first.

The Increasing Savvy of Patients

The world is changing for healthcare, and this is especially true in regard to the nature of the patient/consumer. Clear, compelling communication is central to success, especially in that climate. Yet managers within our industry have not always understood or embraced the value of communication.

That is entirely understandable, as the field of medicine (and correspondingly healthcare) has its roots in the expert model, rather than the consumer-oriented framework that characterized much of American industry in the latter 20th and 21st centuries. The expert, or authority, model—which has its origins in the military—does not follow the creed of "interactive and responsive" feedback but rather is based on the notion that the person in charge has more information at his or her disposal and does not need to solicit input from the individual receiving the direction.

There was a time when the expert model worked quite effectively in the healthcare field. However, society (especially in the developed world) has transformed the nature of healthcare and medicine dramatically. The consumer/patient is much more engaged and informed than ever before and therefore expects—if not demands—interactive communication. In essence, patients want more information, and they want to be more involved in the healthcare experience.

Nothing epitomizes this dynamic more than the rapid rise of the Internet, especially as it relates to accessing healthcare information. As noted by industry futurist, Jeff Goldsmith, "The Internet represents the democratization of American medicine."

In that framework, then, SL communication is crucial to success. Within many hospitals and health systems, the marketing and communications functions are closely linked, if not one and the same. At the very least, both functions often report to the same executive. Consequently, the organization's marketing and communications professionals will need to assess the best means to reach the appropriate audiences and to expend the resources necessary to achieve the determined objectives. This is one of the most important reasons for having marketing and communications staff members participate actively on the SL planning team. Participation will be helpful for them, too, as they can derive great benefit from the clinical experts in regard to the nature of the patient/consumer and the critical audiences involved in the decision process.

For example, in many services, such as cardiology, a solely consumer-directed campaign probably will not prove all that effective, since in most markets the cardiologist decides which hospital or ambulatory setting to use for the procedure or surgery. An effective campaign for cardiology needs to include not only the consumers/patients but also the network of aligned and involved doctors, such as referring (primary care) physicians, internists, cardiologists, and cardiovascular surgeons.

When to Compete, and When to Collaborate

It's easy to fall into the trap of replicating the strategy of the competition. This approach might work in certain cases, but usually it will be viewed as imitative and will be largely ineffective. The notion of "first-mover advantage" holds as true in healthcare as in most other industries; those enterprises that simply follow suit do not often achieve competitive differentiation. Although what the competition is doing is extremely important to consider, it should be only one factor in determining the specific direction of the communication and promotional campaign.

The notion of "first to market"—the idea that the first one to find a position in the consumer's mind is not easily dislodged from that position—has proven its validity over time. More often than not, first place really is the best, and best by a long distance when it comes to perception.

Many times, a marketing approach that merely imitates, or just slightly deviates from, an entrenched competitor's position will actually do more to support the competition than to supplant it. Therefore, the organization that is coming late to the market with a modified approach or a new service establish perceptual ground on which it can differentiate its services and position its uniqueness in the market. Here again is where the application of market research can be highly effective in finding those pockets of differentiation.

Value may also be found in collaboration, rather than in outright competition. This is increasingly true as physicians and hospitals find themselves doing battle with each other more and more frequently. Savvy hospital executives finally are beginning to realize that *aligning* with the doctors may be much more valuable than maligning and going head-to-head with them. Physicians have also begun to realize there may be added value and inherent market advantage in pursuing a collaborative course, as noted previously. Consequently, prior to initiating a full-throttle marketing barrage against the competition (especially if that competition is a multi-physician clinic or another niche player), investigate collaboration, consolidation, or partnership strategies.

Promotion and Positioning

There is a maxim in marketing that states that an individual can be moved only so far within his or her perceptual boundaries. In other words, it is difficult—if not impossible—to move people's perception more than a few degrees in a short time frame. Therefore, it's helpful to know where people's perceptions are. That is one of the greatest benefits of thorough market research: It can help determine the position of an organization's services in the mind of consumers or key stakeholders (such as physicians).

For example, if Hospital A is the widely perceived market leader for oncology services, and Hospital B starts promoting itself as the market leader in oncology, people will not shift their perceptions simply in response to a promotional campaign. In fact, Hospital B will actually foster Hospital A's image and awareness by taking that approach.

Prior to launching a major educational or promotional endeavor that focuses on raising awareness and cementing SL position, it is absolutely essential that the organization assess its positioning in the public's mind. The fact is that in many cases, when asked which hospital provides the highest quality, best physicians, or greatest value, many people respond, "I don't know." This was the feedback received by a multi-hospital system in Texas that conducted its research among more than 800 people in the metropolitan area. Of the six SL areas surveyed to determine people's top-of-mind awareness and general preferences, more than 50% of the people answered "don't know" for five of the six SLs. Unless they've had experience with a particular SL, many consumers admit that they don't have the background or available information to assess which hospital offers the "best" or highest quality at the SL level.

These "don't know" survey results usually mean that the prime perceptual position is up for grabs, given a reasonable and believable message, especially if the organizations have a generally solid reputation overall. But that perceptual position will also be derived from the overall reputation of the hospital or health system, which is not easily modified.

Consider this example, from several years ago. One small community hospital in the Pacific Northwest began billing itself as the market leader in cardiology services. This was a tactical mistake, as the competition in the area was a highly respected, tertiary provider of care. The smaller hospital would have been wiser to focus on an SL (e.g., women's services) that didn't imply the need for the advanced technology and greater resources required by cardiology and more readily identified with the larger hospital. In essence, by laying claim to a market position that did not sync up with the organizational perception, the small community hospital was actually promoting its competition.

The other key thing to keep in mind in terms of promoting an SL or a particular clinical area within a hospital or health system is to ensure that the service promised and the care delivered meet the expectations created by the promotional effort. If a facility overpromises and then under delivers, even though it may derive a short-term benefit (from increased awareness and perhaps some additional volume), the long-range disconnect between wind-up pitch and actual delivery will cause more harm than good.

This is especially true today, when people are much more healthcare savvy due to the Internet and the effort to develop public data report cards. The curtains are gradually being pulled back, and people are increasingly interested in assessing what is actually happening—from a quality standpoint—at the facilities where they send their loved ones or where they are admitted themselves. Consequently, the message delivered must be consistent with the quality available and reported…and the experience received.

Innovative Market Maneuvers

Along with the more traditional venues for outpatient delivery, we also are seeing innovative and atypical venues emerge in the industry. As we've discussed, retail medicine is emerging rapidly as a viable prospect for many systems and individual hospitals. And the avenues for high-tech application of inventive approaches are proving to be popular and effective.

A case in point is the central coordination of ICU stations, wherein an intensivist operates like an air traffic controller, monitoring patients who are often at several disparate locations—from one central monitor. This type of innovation offers both a means of differentiation as well as possible resource efficiency. Although each organization must assess its own readiness and need for innovative venues and approaches, creative applications of this sort will only intensify over the next few years. With the rise of telemedicine, mobile apps, and home-based treatment, the resulting technical and system innovation will engender a delivery model much different than what we've experienced over the decades—and what we're experiencing right now.

Many of the items described in the preceding paragraphs could be considered areas for product development, and indeed they are. Yet there are myriad opportunities for such development in this field right now. There are a few consulting firms (some quite prominent) whose sole focus is keeping healthcare executives apprised of the latest and greatest equipment and technology for particular SLs.

Pursuing the very latest technology can be a tempting and expensive approach—and it can prove both frustrating and financially disappointing. Many within our industry might think this critical assessment is the purview or stewardship of the operational experts, but you should consider enlisting the marketing professionals as well. As mentioned earlier, marketing staff members can assist an organization in assessing not only the perceptual fit of new technology with key audiences (including physicians) but also the level of comfort and message resonance with the purchasing and consuming audiences.

For example, a rural hospital with a mediocre reputation may not benefit that much by installing the latest surgical technology, as the expense may outweigh the benefit, and—as in the example of the small community hospital noted above making a play in a subspecialty area—the consumer/patient may not connect the hospital's current perceptual placement with its desired future position. Even more important, the mystique of the latest high-tech treatments and devices has proven to be somewhat of a medical mirage in more than a few cases, where sometimes the quality is no better than the previous approach.

All the components and characteristics previously mentioned—including market research—can be factored into the consideration and acquisition of new products of SL extensions. For example, even though some hospital executives might balk at spending a few thousand dollars to conduct focus group research concerning a new service or technology for an established SL, that cost pales in comparison to the extensive funds likely to be expended in bringing the new service or technology on line, not to mention the vast investment at stake if the new offering fails to sync with physician demands and consumer expectations. In other words, it's easier to invest $20,000 on market research before incorporating the latest idea or device into the SL than it is to justify why you spent several million dollars without testing the waters first, only to find that the "innovation" that you offered up was the medical equivalent of the Ford Edsel.

Conclusion

Marketing and its related functions and applications have achieved such success in other industries that it is somewhat disquieting to realize how little credence it is given in healthcare. Marketing is the functional engine behind much of America's success in industry.

The SL construct provides healthcare organizations with the framework to tap into the skills and inherent expertise of the marketing model. As stated many times throughout this book, although the SL solution should not be considered merely the domain of marketing, professionals within the function can use its focus on consumers and market responsiveness to assist the organization in meeting its goals and becoming a market-driven system or hospital. That kind of market-facing acumen and adroitness are needed now more than ever in this field, and it resides largely within the marketing domain, and under its direction.

13

Second-Stage SL Execution

Rightsizing the Portfolio

Even though the healthcare industry has employed the service line (SL) model for nearly three decades, there still are organizational leaders who are locked into the old construct of trying to provide all services to all people. Although more executives have realized the folly of that strategy over the past several years, there are still too many who fail to employ the basic business mantra of "sizing to fit" the needs of the key stakeholders and the reimbursement structure of the market.

Given the fleet-footed, retail-oriented competition base that is emerging, healthcare organizations need to conduct a rigorous, objective assessment or "audit" of the organizational position and develop a strategic approach to align its portfolio with the interests and needs of their individual markets. This is a new day in healthcare; the old commitment to providing "all services to all people" is a recipe for mediocre performance at best and outright failure eventually.

Assessing or 'Auditing' the Existing Structure

Here are some questions to ask relative to the enterprise model and its existing portfolio of services:

- Does the portfolio of services and offerings reflect the current and emerging competition, new market forces, and changing physician attitudes? For example, is the organization still providing a SL that is losing ground competitively or technologically, experiencing dramatic economic challenges in the market, or in decline generally, such as obstetrics services?

- Is the current portfolio/operational framework meeting its stated goal of helping the organization become more agile and responsive to changing consumer demands and shifting market forces?

- Has the organizational model been embraced by all key stakeholder groups within the organization? If not, what is required to make that happen?

- Are the individuals in charge of your SL efforts the kind of entrepreneurial leaders who will recognize and act on opportunities to keep the organization on the vanguard of healthcare strategy?

- Are the executive team and board of directors mindful and appreciative of the potential of a robust SL strategy and the significance that the SL model can play in sustaining the organization's long-range mission?

- Are the executive team and board of directors committed to backing service line management (SLM) with sufficient resources, managerial oversight, and long-term execution?

These and other difficult questions should be posed within each organization that wants to succeed in SLM. If the answers you receive indicate that the senior leadership team feels it has not moved the needle much in terms of adapting the SL model and the portfolio of services to the current environment, then step back and consider what must happen to update the model and the strategic approach.

On the other hand, if the leadership team feels that the existing SL model is in fact streamlined, robust, and substantive, then the organization can move forward with its execution of the SLs under consideration and apply the principles throughout the entire enterprise, beyond the three or four lines selected in the first implementation stage of the SL model.

Hardwiring the process for second-stage SLs

Once the organization has effectively proven out the SL model with its existing portfolio of three or four key/core services lines and demonstrated success by achieving the identified metrics over a two- to three-year period, then the framework can be applied to other SLs within the organization. This second stage of SL implementation is important: The concept of an SL strategy must eventually be pervasive throughout the organization. There should be buy-in for the concept at all levels and throughout all departments and functions. If there is not, the model is not likely to deliver its full potential.

One of the fundamental problems with the first wave of SLM implementation in healthcare (back in the mid- to late eighties) was a lack of organizational buy-in. SLM was viewed as the sole purview and responsibility of the marketing department, and, consequently, it failed to deliver its full value because it didn't receive the resources, attention, or cooperation needed from other departments.

Common mistakes to avoid

To that end, once the organization has developed and successfully executed the framework on the core SLs, it can move forward with a more expanded SL implementation, extending the SL model to the second tier of SLs. These SLs typically offer lower growth and lower margins than the core three or four SLs, and might include SLs like general medicine, nephrology, urology, pediatrics, and so forth. This second-stage implementation can (and should) be done gradually; once again following the basic steps outlined in this book for the first-stage SLs. For example, metrics that originally were developed and adopted to determine the SLs in first stage should be used to identify the next one, two, or three SLs that will receive the organization's next level of attention and resources.

The key is to *proceed incrementally*. Most organizations that have attempted to implement or institute an SL approach unsuccessfully have experienced frustration or outright failure for three main reasons:

1. **General misunderstanding of the SL concept.** As noted several times throughout this book, if the SL structure and execution are left up to the marketing professionals and solely within the purview of their department, I can pretty much guarantee a suboptimal execution, if not outright failure. It has to be as operational in nature as it is strategic in execution, or it will never get off the ground.

2. **Unrealistic expectations in terms of how quickly the model can produce results and provide market differentiation**. Implementing a refined SL model is neither a quick fix nor a panacea; it is a data-driven, market-oriented, and business-savvy approach to focusing on the services that resonate most with patients/consumers and that matter most for the organization's success. In essence, these services reflect the organization at its best and therefore have the greatest likelihood of long-term performance against competitors.

3. **Attempting to do too much too fast**. Like other large-scale organizations, hospitals and health systems are complex. Arguably, they are more complex than other enterprises of similar size, due to the multiple stakeholders, the extreme level of regulation, and the convoluted financing architecture. In a sense, they are like supertankers—and supertankers do not change course easily or rapidly. Consequently, in implementing an SL strategy, incremental adoption and application are more likely to succeed than an organizationwide, all-encompassing adoption of the model.

For these reasons and others, even after success has been achieved with the three or four core SLs, it's better to apply the SL model to additional lines incrementally. The additional SLs that are identified should be second-tier (not bottom of the ladder), as they still must represent high-priority categories or strategic business units that will help the organization maintain sustainability and ensure long-range financial viability.

Implementing the Second Stage

The second-stage SL process is fundamentally the same as the first phase. You'll find that the second tier of SL implementation (important SLs that are less critical to the organization's long-range success) should be easier to implement than the first group, since the difficult pioneering work already is accomplished.

However, resist the temptation to use the greater ease of implementation as justification for immediately identifying and implementing an additional five or six SLs. You and those charged with second-stage SL implementation will still face issues of political barriers, physician alignment, resource allocation, and territoriality that come with all functions and nearly all organizations. Consequently, the second stage should involve no more than one to three additional SLs.

The newly identified SL managers and supporting matrix teams (for the second phase) can learn much from their now-experienced counterparts, but they still have a fairly difficult road ahead to incorporate the planning, principles, and discipline of the SL model.

Downsizing the organization's portfolio of services

Another valuable outcome that should emerge from applying the processes in this book is a fundamental **streamlining** of the organization and continuous trimming of its portfolio of services. This pruning can occur organically as you identify marginally producing SLs.

One of the most challenging dilemmas that healthcare executives must face is what to do with marginally performing SLs. Based on the track record of many health systems (and hospitals), it is quite obvious that as an industry we are not particularly comfortable with rightsizing the portfolio.

The danger of delaying action: A case study

One example of the potential downside of not asking the difficult questions nor confronting the need to right size the portfolio occurred in a nonprofit hospital system in the Southern United States. This particular hospital system purchased three urgent care medical clinics a few years ago. These clinics had been started by a doctor and a business partner and were marginally successful. The clinics were purchased at a time when the hospital was looking to expand its outreach efforts, integrate better with the physicians, and increase its overall market share.

In the first few years, the clinics proved to be a good diversification for the system. Even though financially they didn't do much better than breakeven, they increased awareness of the health system and improved accessibility for patients. Over time, though, changes in the local managed-care reimbursement structure caused the clinics to exhibit declining financial performance and become more of a monetary drain.

Despite this deteriorating situation, the executive responsible for the clinics and the physician who had started them adamantly opposed putting the sale or closure option for the clinics on the table. These two leaders consistently maintained that shutting down the clinics simply was not an option worth considering.

By refusing to outline options for the poor-performing clinics, including the most dramatic alternative—namely to shutter the operations--in their discussions with senior leaders, they limited their options and, in essence, skewed the evaluation of the clinics' true conditions. In so doing, they failed to provide an objective performance assessment. Eventually, the system closed the clinics in an 11th-hour, rushed fashion which was off-putting for virtually all the parties involved, from the physicians employed by the clinics to the patients who relied on those enterprises for their care. Such is the risk of delaying a difficult, but data-based and market-oriented portfolio assessment and putting all options on the table, including the possibility of closure.

In other industries, the trimming of service or product offerings is one of the most vital functions a successful management team can undertake. In fact, the hallmark of most successful organizations is an ability to determine when to de-market (scale back on marketing and promotional efforts), consolidate, or jettison altogether poorly performing segments of the portfolio.

In our industry, the reluctance to jettison services is understandable for a couple of reasons. First, the healthcare field's origins lie in a *cost-reimbursed financial rubric*. Consequently, paring down the portfolio by eliminating services was just not even an element of the business model in the early decades of the industry.

In fact, for many decades, the managerial approach was to bulk up the service offerings so as to increase the base on which reimbursement could be made. This approach changed with the implementation of prospective payment and the overriding need for greater efficiency. While most of that sentiment has vanished over the last couple decades, the old-school managerial mind set still lingers in some executive suites. Yet to prevail in a much more competitive environment that demands constant assessment of the organization's portfolio, we must shift our thinking and transform our approach.

Even more pervasive than the cost-reimbursed financial bias is the notion that hospitals must provide *all services to all people*. Understandably, this belief stems from the model of a community hospital offering comprehensive services to the residents within its geographic reach. Although this attitude and approach are admirable from a philosophical standpoint, from a business enterprise vantage, this model is no longer sustainable for most organizations.

Determining value to the market

We live in a world of specialization, and healthcare is not immune to that reality. Consequently, hospital and health system leaders must be vigilant in their managerial responsibility and community stewardship to ensure that the services their organizations provide are both *valued by the market* and contributing to the financial stability of the organization.

To determine value to the market, this question must be posed to whatever forces, groups, or individuals are paying (reimbursing) for the service: *Does the revenue exceed the expenses to provide the service?* If not, each executive team must ask itself, "Why are we providing this service?" The market is sending a message that the service in question is not worth the cost to provide it.

In other industries, this type of negative market response to reimbursement for products or services would be cause for immediate evaluation, possible recalibration, and—if the service can't be rendered operationally profitable—the likely termination of the services in question. Obviously, in the healthcare field, it's more complex than that, but the underlying rationale and element of fiscal reasoning is basically the same, or at least should be.

In the case of marginally performing SLs, the senior leaders and SL managers and directors should pose questions such as the following:

- Are our costs out of line, or is this a marketwide reality?

- Are we receiving appropriate (and market-comparable) reimbursement for these services—from managed care, government, employers, or other payers?

- Does the current setting for the delivery of this service offer optimal efficiency? (For example, consider that the nature of reimbursement may have basically "dictated" that this service shift to an outpatient setting.)

- Has this service moved beyond its expected value equivalent or, in other words, is it still viable given economic realities?

- Is there an opportunity to consolidate with other services or collaborate with other providers?

- Are key organizational players aware of the financial drain of these services on overall economics and the ramifications for the long-term viability of the enterprise?

- What kind of fallout would we experience from key stakeholder groups if we diminish, consolidate, or discontinue this SL?

These are difficult questions to ask and challenging options to consider. Nonetheless, each organization should regularly ask these and similar questions about marginal SLs. The exercise of identifying and discussing marginal SLs will prove illuminating for senior leaders and governance bodies of organizations that follow the process. Ultimately, such an effort will likely prove worthwhile for the community as well.

As highlighted in the urgent care case study presented earlier in this chapter, some system leaders are hesitant to start down the path of analysis, as they dread the outcome and reaction to possible elimination of SLs. Despite that fear, consolidation or elimination of SLs should always be on the table. It needn't be the final selection, but by considering the option of discontinuation as a possibility, the overall evaluation of the SL will be more forthright and honest.

Some people believe that putting an option on the table makes it the only solution, and many people gravitate to the most drastic alternative. In a few isolated enterprises, that may be the case, but in most organizations, based on my observation, it is not. Furthermore, providing the full range of alternatives— including closure—establishes an important managerial tenet, namely that no project is so sacrosanct or off limits that it should not be evaluated objectively and comprehensively.

Women's services: To OB or not to OB

Several years ago, I received a call from a colleague in consulting who had been engaged by a hospital to assess the viability of that facility's obstetric (OB) services. He asked me if I had any reservations in shutting down the OB SL. Without much hesitation, I responded, "Probably not a good idea, given the fact that for many women, the birthing experience is their first adult encounter with a hospital." He thanked me, hung up, and called another colleague for a second opinion.

If I were asked the same question now, I would probably give a very different answer. Times have changed, reimbursement has shifted, and patient loyalty is not what it once was. What a difference a decade makes. In fact, one mid-size for-profit system evaluated the OB services in each of its hospitals for profitability and long-term viability and, as part of that assessment, decided to shut down several OB departments.

A large faith-based system in the upper-Midwest made a similar determination with one of its hospitals that had the lowest number of births in a three-hospital town. Even though birthing services were an integral part of the "caring from birth to death" mission/mantra of this system, they reasoned that since the services were available in the community with two competitive high-quality facilities, they needed to make a market-need and financially based decision to close the unit. It was not an easy decision, but on several levels, it was arguably the right one to make.

Adhering to the principle that nothing is above full scrutiny, based on empirical assessment (and not tradition-bound parameters or prominent-figure dispensations), also demonstrates that management is willing to constantly and meticulously evaluate all levels of the operation in an effort to monitor and improve. Fundamentally, portfolio analysis is sound stewardship—nothing more, nothing less.

The point is that an SL approach offers one of the most definitive managerial structures for assessing marginal lines and then for determining options to deal with such areas of operation. On an individual service segment basis, the marginally performing areas can be assigned to SL managers and teams, with accountability for improving performance directly on their shoulders.

Conclusion

Once the organization has successfully incorporated an SL model into its operating structure and has realized initial success with a few core SLs (those first identified as the highest priority), it then can transition gradually and thoughtfully into identifying an additional (but still limited) number of other SLs for the SLM model. This approach and application should follow the same pattern and steps as were used for the inaugural three or four core SLs.

Another key characteristic and benefit of the SL model is its ability to identify and isolate those lines that are marginal performers. This analysis can and should be completed early in the overall process, when the SLs are ranked based on the metrics the organization has identified as the key elements for long-term success. Once the marginal lines are identified, the organization periodically should evaluate, discuss, and determine the best option for handling these lesser performers. These options include de-marketing (scaling back on promotion, resource allocation, and managerial time), consolidation, collaboration with other providers, and discontinuance altogether. Obviously, the latter option should be considered carefully in light of the response of key stakeholders, the reaction of the community, and the impact of discontinuance on other SLs in the enterprise individually and within the context of the overall organization. All that noted, a well-considered decision to eliminate or dramatically reduce poor-performing SLs will prove to be one of the most important decisions senior leaders make and one of the most beneficial strategies the organization executes.

Afterword

Seizing Share under Accountable Care

The healthcare industry faces a maelstrom of market forces that are producing and will continue to produce tectonic change and unprecedented disruption. This is not necessarily a bad thing. In fact, a fair number of industry observers would likely argue that we are long overdue; our spending on healthcare is unreasonable and unsustainable. These observers might go on to add that the value for our colossal investment simply is not there—at least by comparison to other industrialized nations which spend far less and arguably provide far more.

It's clear that the shift from the old model to a new one is necessary and probably beneficial, though only time will tell that story. A number of pundits have referred to this shift—the move away from a fee-for-service model to accountable care and bundled payments—as transitioning from "volume to value." While that phrase is useful, it doesn't capture the nature of the consumer-focused dynamic at hand, which provides the underpinning of our shift from episodic care to population health.

To sharpen our focus on the true locus of change, I describe our metamorphosis not in terms of changes to what we provide (volume is replaced by value), but in terms of the individuals who use our services. We are in essence transforming our delivery model emphasis from the acutely ill to the astutely well. And that is nothing short of a seismic shift.

Given this dynamic, which at its core involves such a massive re-envisioning, repurposing and recalibration of our fundamental approach to providing health services, we need to pull up and assess the vantage from which this redefinition and reinvention of our model should occur. I would recommend that the lens though which this change should be revisited and revised is that of the consumer/patient. Finally, we have the opportunity to fully engage the end user of the services we provide and now—given the emerging shift in payment responsibility and methodology—the ultimate "payer" as well.

If one accepts that premise, then what better framework or construct to accurately represent the consumer/patient then that of service line architecture? This approach is arguably the most reliable and empirically-established model for aligning with consumer interests, wants, and needs. The very nature of a service line construct—with its emphasis on market research, competitive reconnaissance, manager accountability and defined business objectives—provides a consumer-centric, market-based mosaic that few other models or frameworks begin to approach.

In the case of healthcare services in the 21st century, the two converging forces of rising consumerism and an emerging population health framework provide further substantiation that a service line focus is both a fitting solution to the changing dynamic we are experiencing in the health sector and (arguably) the solution to meeting and addressing the dramatic changes we face now and can expect over the next several years.

The necessary shift in focus from the acutely ill to the astutely well is almost tailor made for an SL orientation, since our new perspective embodies the very principles discussed throughout this book and aligns perfectly with the fundamental, consumer-aware steps to instituting a successful service line approach, including everything from defining the service lines to developing rigorous business plans to achieve the organization's objectives as they relate to each strategic business unit of the enterprise.

Our industry's colossal shift away from an expert model to a consumer-driven construct demand that we understand the consumer/patient at a level that we could not have imagined in the past. We must take a much more sophisticated and dedicated approach to analytics, predictive modeling, and the general application of "big data." We must develop an in-depth understanding of behavioral science and apply that understanding to tapping the vast opportunities that field represents in terms of modeling, predicting, and influencing behavior. Applications such as "gamification" offer the potential to modify behavior under a population health model, and will not only be explored in the next few years, I predict that they will be employed significantly and effectively.

Other industries have mastered the art and science of understanding the consumer and applying leading-edge technology and acumen to that endeavor. The healthcare industry must follow.